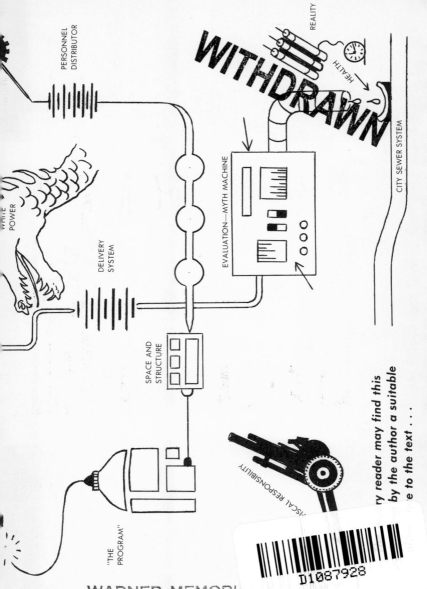

WITHDRAWN

PERSONNEL DISTRIBUTOR

REALITY

HEALTH

WHITE POWER

CITY SEWER SYSTEM

DELIVERY SYSTEM

EVALUATION—MYTH MACHINE

SPACE AND STRUCTURE

"THE PROGRAM"

FISCAL RESPONSIBILITY

...ry reader may find this
...by the author a suitable
...e to the text . . .

D1087928

COMMUNITY MENTAL HEALTH
Myth and Reality

COMMUNITY MENTAL HEALTH

Myth and Reality

ANTHONY F. PANZETTA, M.D.
Associate Professor of Psychiatry
Temple University
Philadelphia, Pennsylvania

Foreword by
C. KNIGHT ALDRICH, M.D.

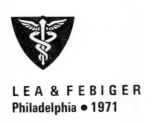

LEA & FEBIGER
Philadelphia • 1971

ISBN 0−8121−0358−0
Library of Congress Catalog Card Number: 71−152029
Published in Great Britain by Henry C. Kimpton Publishers, London
Printed in the United States

TO DR. JOHN ROMANO,
a wise and scholarly teacher who practiced community psychiatry
before it was fashionable.

FOREWORD

Seven and a half years—less than the span of two Presidential terms—have passed at this writing since the enactment of Public Law 88-164 catapulted community psychiatry out of the theoretical and pilot stage and into a national program. This law, backed by mental health professionals and others with perhaps more enthusiasm than experience, promised the resources with which to plan, build, and man the means of total national implementation of social psychiatry's theory.

Massive, abrupt implementation of relatively untried theory that catches the legislators' fancy is the American style. In our efforts to change society, we do not take easily to the slow, conservative process of evolution from theory to practice through controlled experiment or trial and error; for the most part, the results of the experiments we do support are ignored. We want action, on a broad front, whether in industry, in the military or in health, education and welfare. We want action, and we want results, and if results are not apparent and apparent soon, we are tempted impatiently to abandon the whole idea, particularly if it has been associated with a previous administration.

The program envisioned by Public Law 88-164, if carried through, would ultimately have resulted in 2,000 community mental health centers, providing comprehensive and accessible prevention and early treatment services to every U.S. citizen. It was—and still is—an ambitious program, broad in scope and difficult to evaluate. But after an initial flurry of activity, the pace has become much slower; construction and staffing are behind schedule, and there is some question whether centers now in the planning stage will be funded, or even whether centers already built or under construction will be staffed, at least in the patterns laid out by the composers of 88-164.

What will happen to community mental health centers in the next eight years? Will the program be abandoned; will the centers continue to multiply? Will they come to resemble more conventional clinics; or will they be absorbed into community or neighborhood health centers? Their future depends on a multitude of political, economic and philosophical factors, many of which are intimately related to emerging patterns of distribution of general health care. If the program survives, whether or not the centers retain their autonomy and identity, a closer tie to the rest of medicine seems inevitable.

Community mental health centers may, in fact, be unwitting testing grounds for an even broader program of community care involving not just one medical specialty but all of medicine. Whatever their fate, but particularly if indeed they are destined to serve as pilots for future community health centers, they require the most careful critical evaluation, critical evaluation that is not limited to the "hard" data of cost accounting and of indices of incidence and prevalence, but includes the richer, more subjective "soft" data that are obtained from appraisals by participants and observers. In evaluating any social institution, historical data from those most intimately involved are needed.

This book is an evaluation of the community mental health center program, derived from personal observations of a key member of a community mental health center family. Dr. Panzetta, after four years in the midst of his center's activities, took time off to reflect, and to gain perspective for generalizing from his experience. He has written neither an attack on, nor a defense of, community mental health centers or the community mental health "movement." Instead, he has written a thoughtful and challenging appraisal of where we stand today, in 1971, with respect to the nation's response to the concern which led to the Joint Congressional Commission on Mental Illness and Health and its report, "Action for Mental Health." In his critique of the consequences of Public Law 88-164, he is concerned with such fundamental questions as: Is the concept of "community," so basic to the Community Mental Health Center Act, applicable to today's cities? Is the "catchment area" a rational basis on which to decentralize health services? Can a community be "organized" for such an idiosyncratic and esoteric service as mental health? Is a truly "comprehensive" mental health service possible or feasible? What does prevention of mental illness really require? Can quality control be introduced into community mental health operations? Has role diffusion been overdone in community psychiatry staffing? Is the community mental health movement overcommitted to social reform? What are the consequences of providing power to the community without community responsibility?

These crucial questions must be considered seriously if the community mental health movement is to make the most of its potentialitites as a continuing influence on the nation's mental health, as a pilot for planners and organizers of community health centers, or even solely as an historical phenomenon.

Dr. Panzetta's answers to these questions are provocative and unconventional as well as thoughtful. Whether one agrees with him or not, however, it is important to those concerned with the future of community mental health or community health seriously to consider the views and conclusions and predictions he presents on the following pages.

C. Knight Aldrich

PREFACE

This book is intended for those stout souls who contemplate a career in "community mental health" or "community psychiatry," or for those weary souls who may be about to leave such a career. It may also prove of value to those who are already expert in the field, whether by experience, intuition, or revelation. Although the text is often addressed to the psychiatrist, anyone within community mental health will be conversant with the material and may find it of some value. Community mental health has proven to be a haven for many "mental health" disciplines, as well as for the undisciplined.

Although the reader may anticipate a critical devaluation, I will make a strong disclaimer at the outset. It is precisely because I believe in the fundamental worth of the community mental health movement that I am compelled to write this book. In the warp and woof of any "movement," a good deal of unnecessary and immature noise is generated. It seems periodically necessary to dissect those elements of pretension and tinsel from those of worth.

I have been impressed by the numerous and lofty books written about community psychiatry and community mental health but more impressed by their distance from reality. I thought that a book written about the travail in this field might be helpful. Although I am prone to making sweeping generalizations, I have just survived four years of specific experience and I have tried to temper the generalization with the primary data of that experience.

I liken myself to a frontiersman in a way. On the heels of the federal enabling legislation, I began a four year odyssey in an urban community mental health center. The center was "innovative," "bold," and at the cutting edge of the community psychiatry movement. Issues presented themselves in raw perspective and, because of our predisposition to error, we not only learned about "how to" but very often "how not to."

The frontiersman of the Old West, in many ways, was a sacrificial offering for the subsequent development of that area. History might see his role as experimenter in ways of surviving. He had little experience to call upon and little ability to anticipate all of the challenges he would face. Armed with his convictions and ignorance he laid ground for his followers. So too, the role of the community psychiatrist is predictably sacrificial and transitional.

During my psychiatric residency at the University of Rochester, I spent a six-month elective in the Division of Preventive and Community Psychiatry. This was a new program within the Department and was directed by Dr. Elmer Gardner who had launched a highly successful register study in Monroe County. With the epidemiologic potential of the register study, this Division was undertaking broad based studies within the County and was also developing consultation programs to community institutions such as the courts, police, social agencies, and homes for the aged. The value of such activity seemed self-evident to me and was exciting and gratifying. When I left Rochester to begin a two-year service commitment in the U.S. Navy, I realized that my career plans would have to include the orientation to community institutions that I had experienced during that six-month elective.

My two-year experience at the United States Naval Hospital in Philadelphia reinforced my appreciation for working with patients within a broader system context. The ability to influence the system in the interest of the patient was limited but nonetheless it was clear that patient's behavior was not simply a function of internal dynamics.

When my discharge time drew near (July 1966) I was certain that I would have to work in a situation that could allow me to pursue my interest in synthesizing intrapsychic and socio-cultural determinants of behavior. I felt that both were necessary in understanding human behavior and I was aware of the lack of synthesis between these approaches. It was troubling to hear the dialogue between their adherents take on a partisan and provincial quality. The back and forth derision did little to help a young psychiatrist trying to settle into his first responsible career assignment after the military. It was this need to clarify my decision to myself that led to the writing of the paper "Causal and Action Models in Social Psychiatry" (Archives of General Psychiatry, March 1967). A modified version of that paper is included in this book as Chapter 8.

And then came an unexpected opportunity. Dr. Elmer Gardner had decided to leave Rochester and was coming to Temple University in Philadelphia. Plans were still vague at that time but he was going to develop a Community and Social Psychiatry program and he invited me to join him. The plans then crystalized abruptly as it became clear that Community Mental Health Centers were to be "the way" for community or social minded psychiatrists. Three of my colleagues from the Rochester residency had also been invited to join Dr. Gardner and the prospect of the four of us working together with Dr. Gardner was enough to make me decide to become a community psychiatrist—Philadelphia style.

The early phase was exciting and heady. There was much to be learned about the community around Temple University in North Philadelphia and much to be learned about what community psychiatry meant. The community mental health center was a new structure for all of us, but gratefully it was spelled out to some degree in the requirements for specific services and programs. Little did I realize then that the clarity that seemed to flow from those requirements would prove to be illusory in the long run.

Dr. Gardner, as Director of the Community Mental Health Center, began an energetic recruitment program for further staff and we four "charter associates," as it were, each took responsibility for various program parts. Dr. Louis Harris was to head our in-patient program. Dr. Fred Glaser was to head our partial hospitalization program. Dr. William Hetznecker was to head our children and family program. I was to head the emergency program. We seemed to have a rather clear mandate, we were given enormous freedom and responsibility, and financial resource for staff was ample. The University and the Department of Psychiatry gave us a green light and vigorous support.

Recruitment went very well and we began attracting professional staff with competence and energy. The elan of those early days was high and everyone felt that we were in pursuit of noble goals and that we had resources to achieve those goals. Each of the four "charter associates" went about the complicated task of building their own part of the center. We shared one another's dreams, plans, problems and frustration but more significantly, we each became preoccupied with our own unit. This seemed reasonable at the time since each unit had a large task before it and we felt justified in building the pieces before putting them together.

The rate of our development was gratifying. We came to Temple in August of 1966 and by the Spring of 1967 we had begun our clinical services and by that summer we were totally operative. From an assortment of ideas and commitment we had erected a fully operating community mental health center within a year. We were proud and ready for more. The impression that we were on the right track seemed further supported by the interest being paid us from many quarters. N.I.M.H. considered us a model center, or so we believed, and visitors came to Philadelphia from around the country. Each part of our Center's program bore its own individuality and uniqueness. The emergency service, called the Crisis Center, was in a row house, and the staff was seeing walk-ins and police cases. It was the only bona-fide twenty-four hour per day psychiatric emergency service in Philadelphia which had no rigid policy of exclusion. The out-patient service, called the Psychosocial Clinic, was also in a neighborhood row house and it tried working without a waiting list. It used indigenous non-professionals as primary therapists and was without precedent in its bold approach. The partial-hospitalization service, a day program called "Our Place," developed a unique therapeutic community format with patients and staff attempting to disregard their hierarchical status. Resocialization became their therapeutic goal. The children and family program was organized around consultative and educational input to schools and to the Center staff. The in-patient service was willingly and planfully located in a State Hospital so that we could not avoid responsibility for our patients.

The gaps between the services were becoming more apparent as time went on but we could look to our immediate gains and urge patience from those who would comment on our limitations.

There were many critics, of course. Some were within our organization and some were outside. The latter critics, particularly those from the social agencies of the city, were at times indignant about our use of non-professional therapists. Our colleagues from the academic scene were also periodically upset and at times appalled at our brashness. All in all, however, we were able to hold our own in these encounters and our rationale for our programs was, if not convincing, at least understandable.

The morale of staff seemed high at first. Everyone seemed eager to show our critics that they were wrong. There was also an intoxicating feeling that came from knowing you were "where the action was." The urban dilemma, the crisis of the city, the black revolution, poverty and mental illness, the culture of the deprived . . . racism, political power, change agents, prevention . . . all of these rally concepts seemed to be part of our intravenous diet.

But within our bubbling pot, many issues began to surface, each with its own cadre of advocates. Some wanted the Center to pursue social goals, others wanted the Center to pursue clinical goals, others wanted both, others wanted to restrict goals to very few, others to very many.

The problem of racism, so well demonstrated in the society at large, was inching into our organizational awareness. How much was there?—where was it?—who had it?—against whom?—why? The Center became introspective. Meetings turned into group therapy. Insights turned into accusations.

As we went on, the inevitable burden of our patient's problems grew heavier. The multiple problem family, so neatly described in the antiseptic pages of our journals, were everywhere. A patient was simply the emerged part of an enormous iceberg of family and societal disturbances. The handle to a case proved to be an illusion. Therapy, whether provided by the expert professional or the

minimally trained non-professional, was the euphemism
for anemic handwringing.

With all of this going on simultaneously, it was no
wonder that scapegoating became the order of the day.
Everyone seemed to be part of either an accusatory or
accused group. As with most scapegoating practices, the
targets tended to be among those "in charge." It mattered
little who you were, or how highly placed you were, there
was always someone else above you who was destroying
the whole program.

Eventually our difficulties began to preoccupy time at
the expense of the various programs. Patient care became a
backdrop to the more immediate pressure of internal fragmentation. Fair play committees, staff advisory councils,
plenary staff meetings, all-day meetings and emergency
executive council sessions became routine. Disagreement
gave way to hostility.

The saga of the Temple Community Mental Health
Center could take up the entirety of this book but I shall
resist that temptation. The reader should realize, however,
that the events summarized so globally above took four
years to unfold. It is difficult to know how many lessons
were really learned by our mistakes and how many new
illusions were created. This book attempts to present at
least the lessons learned by me.

Whether my myths and realities measure up to those
listed in the ultimate book of truth is doubtful.

The reader may interpret the affect of the book as being
angry or overly cynical. It would be incorrect for me to
deny that I had deep and perplexing feelings about the
Center. But lessons are often better learned in the heat of
disappointment and frustration than in the glow of
success. I have elected not to extract the feelings from the
words and beg the indulgence of the reader, who would
prefer more pablum and less sauce.

In retrospect it is easy to see how young professionals,

intent on an exciting mission, could take themselves so seriously. It is a major intent of this book to replace the somber perspective attached to community psychiatry with a more realistic appreciation of its value, its major unresolved conceptual and practical problems, and its pretensions.

The chapters are organized around the major issues which faced me during those four years. They touch upon the core of community psychiatry. Some have relevance to other aspects of the psychiatric art. Some are relevant to organizational life in or out of medicine. Some are simply the issues of living one's life in a productive fashion. The experiences which led to the writing of this book are urban in quality. Temple University Community Mental Health Center is located in North Philadelphia, in an area of devastating social chaos. The parameters of social breakdown are at their worst in this "ghetto" and the problems of a mental health center—both in terms of the people to be served, as well as the organizational and developmental issues of the center—stand out in stark relief. In many ways such an experience can serve as a "survival school." Although there are undoubtedly many differences and hence many variations in the quality and quantity of problems faced by various centers in various locales, there are many issues which will obtain regardless of the situation. It is with an eye towards these general issues that this book is written.

There are many people to thank for help in writing this book. Dr. Elmer Gardner provided me with opportunity and responsibility. He introduced me to the field and was truly a pathfinder. My gratitude to him must remain deep and personal. My colleagues and friends, Drs. William Hetznecker, Louis Harris and Fred Glaser, shared the fun and frustration and demonstrated the commitment and competence which often sustained me in dark days. And of course, thanks must be paid to the staff of the Center who taught me far more than I was ever able to teach them.

Particular gratitude is due the staff of the Crisis Center and the Psychosocial Clinic. They were loyal when it was difficult but most loyal to the patients who needed them. Cecil Crowder, John Searight and Rosetta Snipe were indispensable and carried burdens without adequate recognition. Their good cheer and dependability were a rich gift.

I must also thank the Department of Psychiatry at Temple University and its chairman, Dr. R. Bruce Sloane, for having granted me the time to put together my thoughts and to write this book. The manuscript was read and critically analyzed by Drs. John Romano, C. Knight Aldrich, David Goldberg, Max Pepernik and Harriet Aronson. I am grateful to them for their frank and helpful critique and suggestions. I am particularly in debt to Dr. Aldrich who went over the manuscript so very carefully and agreed to write the foreword. Dr. Goldberg brought the sobering view of the English empiricist to his reading of the manuscript and has left me with enough new questions for another book.

I am indebted to Cathy Spraggins and Lillian Brooks for their help in preparation of the manuscript and to Betty Ellis for her navigation of the clerical blockades on my behalf. Finally, I could not have completed the book without my wife's encouragement and final editing.

Philadelphia, Pennsylvania   Anthony F. Panzetta

CONTENTS

chapter 1

CONCEPTS OF COMMUNITY:

Is It a Where, a When or a How?

Certain words have a way of taking on meanings never intended. Words of a high level of abstraction are like that. Because they touch so many diverse phenomena, these abstract terms are both practical and impractical at the same time. "Community" is an example of such a word. It can be applied in a variety of situations and so is versatile as a oneword concept. But it also is prone to multiple connotative meanings and so can be easily misunderstood.[1]

In today's mental health vocabulary, "community" has taken a prominent position. To some it rings a public health note, to others it has a socio-political connotation. It may suggest a neighborhood, a district, or an ethnic grouping. It may generate a mood of warmth and together-

1. Arensberg, C.M., Kimball, S.T.: *Culture and Community*, New York: Harcourt, Brace & World, Inc., 1965.

ness or one of pragmatic association. It has a current mystique, however, which transcends any of the usual denotative or connotative meanings. This is a mystique of value, an inherent sense of goodness attached to the various concepts of community. To be pro-community is to be virtuous; to be anti-community is to be evil. Both assessments precede any attempt to clarify what is meant by "community."

Since "community" is so vital a concept in a movement which presumes to use the term to describe itself, it is necessary for us to start with its critical analysis. We shall consider it first from a sociologic perspective and then as a geographic concept, a temporal concept and as a functional concept. The implications of the popular movement of "community control" will be considered as will the racial issues which confuse the concept of community.

GEMEINSCHAFT AND GESELLSCHAFT

Sociologists have grappled with the concept of community since Comte and philosophers since Plato. It is unlikely that we shall settle on the ultimate choice here. There is a useful distinction for our purposes, however, that was elaborated by Tönnies in his use of the terms "gemeinschaft" and "gesellschaft."[2] A gemeinschaft community is characterized by an implicit bond which relates person to person. Like the extended family, such a community is held together by common values, affection, mutual dependence, respect, and a sense of status hierarchy. There are no formal rules of relationship and the roles of the members of that community are set by the traditions and cultural expectations of the group. This type of community is becoming increasingly rare and

2. Nisbet, R.A.: *The Sociological Tradition,* New York: Basic Books, Inc. 1966.

depends for its existence on a rural or feudal type of social organization.

Today's dominant type of community is "gesellschaft" in nature.[3] This is a developmental fact due in great measure to the growing urbanization of modern society. Here the bonds are formal and explicit. People relate to one another through formulated guidelines or even rules and regulations. Affection and dependence on one another for survival is rarely operative. In the gesellschaft community people come together through formal institutions, like their place of employment, their church or their professional or civic organization. Often great blocks of time are spent in these vertical groupings (in institutions usually away from the area of their home) in contrast to the lesser blocks of time spent in horizontal groupings (in their home neighborhood).

It is the reality of the gesellschaft and the longing for the gemeinschaft which often lead to a misorientation of "community minded" psychiatrists. While it is true that there are territorial commitments which all persons make to their "home," and while it is true that this commitment is apt to carry with it affective and durable qualities,[4] it is anachronistic to program for a form of social organization that no longer exists (gemeinschaft). It would seem much more reasonable to program for the dominant form *i.e.* the gesellschaft. If there are existent gemeinschaft forms in the population, then these can be taken into account, but not to the exclusion of the more prevalent gesellschaft forms.

The visible manifestation of the gemeinschaft approach to community mental health planning is the "catchment area." Here a geographic area is designated as target area and all those who live within the specific boundaries are members of the mythical gemeinschaft. This horizontal

3. Nisbet, R.A., ibid.
4. Ardrey, R.: *The Territorial Imperative,* New York: Atheneum, 1966.

approach to community makes sense from a limited public health point of view because it allows for the assignment of responsibility. But this goal, *i.e.* the fixing of responsibility, is an operational accomplishment and does not speak to the issue of community.

There is a further paradox implicit in this approach. One of the ways a gemeinschaft group is maintained is by a radical provincialism. Remnants of such groups remain in some of the ethnic communities of Chicago and they have been able to maintain this Old World coherence by inbreeding and careful exclusion of cultural values of the pluralistic community around them.[5] They have resisted acculturation to an extent (although the resistance is disappearing rapidly) and so are set apart. The Amish settlements of Pennsylvania and Indiana are better examples of the gemeinschaft community. But again, in all of these examples, the gemeinschaft is preserved by a non-integrative approach to the larger surround. The paradox rests with the black neighborhoods which to some extent have also maintained a gemeinschaft way of life but by enforced exclusion from the larger community. Since many, if not most, of the community mental health centers are in black areas, they are forced to program their services in such a way so as to reinforce the separatist ethos of that area. Although this approach may fit into the plans of the militant black activist, it should be recognized as what it is, a closed market.

A visible remaining example of gemeinschaft living which persists throughout modern society (although under great pressure) is the family. It makes great sense to program for family oriented services since this social form is naturally occurring and durable. But it is possible to pro-

5. In an old traveler's guide to Chicago (Drury, J.: *Chicago In 7 Days*, New York: Robert M. McBride & Co., 1930) the city is presented, in a series of maps, as an amalgam of contiguous ethnic districts such as, Little Sicily, Italian section, Polish section, Greek district, Jewish district, Chinatown etc.

gram for family oriented services without paying a great deal of attention to the horizontal community orientation.

This perspective, which differentiates the vertical (institutional) community from the horizontal (geographic) community and which separates the gesellschaft (formal) relationship from the gemeinschaft (mutual dependent) relationship, can and should clarify some of the inherent difficulties as mental health centers program for their assigned "community" (catchment area).

The resolution of this seeming dilemma lies in the careful application of logical definition. If the overriding consideration is the need for a system which fixes medical and paramedical responsibility, then the catchment area concept may indeed be optimum. But to go further and equate catchment area with "community" is a nonsequitur. If the primary goal is to develop programs which fit the idiosyncrasies of a discrete community, then the catchment area concept is meaningless unless the boundaries of the catchment area coincide with the boundaries of an existing gemeinschaft community. If such a community is identified, then we must realize that our efforts may very well serve to reinforce the separatist and exclusionary character of the gemeinschaft community.

WHERE: Community as catchment area

In a clear way, the catchment area community is a "where" community. Its definition is dependent on street names, buildings and general demography. It can be isolated on a wall map which then becomes an impressive addition to one's office, particularly if there is a war games disposition. Colored pins can point out the structural parts of this community and a sense of "my turf" is quickly established. The basic orienting grid to one's thinking becomes "those people living between Susquehanna and Diamond Streets." The great temptation, is to assume that "those people" are like one another in their sense of community, *i.e.* they share common beliefs, common problems and common aspirations. What in fact is the reality?

There is a commonality which presents itself in the "where" community if that community is sufficiently oppressed. The social indicators of such a community are familiar in language today, *i.e.* high death rates, high infant mortality, dilapidated housing, high crime rates, etc. And so the common factors extracted from such a community become logical targets for intervention. These are the "symptoms" of the "where" community and hence the illusory logical target for the community psychiatrist. But the roots of these "symptoms" are not "where" in their vulnerability. A geographic approach may give topographic clues to what is between these boundaries, but it also fixes you to the out-field when the real action is in the in-field. The dilapidated house on Diamond Street is a complex phenomenon derived from City Hall, the money market, the suburban ethos as well as from events and people within the catchment area. If we choose to define our mental health goals in this grand dimension, we had better not assume a catchment area orientation in our programming.

The analysis of a "where" community is usually written in the language of demography and epidemiology.[6] This defined population approach gives valuable information about the target population but it is important to realize the type of information that is supplied. The information on incidence and prevalence for example is only as good as those criteria used for the identification of a "case." The more abstract these criteria, the more unreliable are the results. Because of the availability of rather discrete criteria for the identification of schizophrenia, it has be-

6. Demography is the statistical study of human populations especially with reference to size and density, distribution, and vital statistics. Epidemiology is the science that deals with the incidence, prevalence, distribution and control of disease in a population.

come a favorite object of epidemiologic study,[7] and the results of such studies have a higher degree of validity than studies of more diffusely defined conditions, such as the Mid-Town Manhattan Study.[8]

The point of all this should be clarified here. If a community is defined in "where" terms, its analysis, *i.e.* the dissection of its "problems," is biased in the direction of measurable and gross phenomena. What emerges is a picture of the social disorder of that area as reflected in incidence and prevalence rates of the high visibility problems. Programming for the "where" community will therefore inevitably tend towards these high visibility problems. This may or may not correspond with planning objectives derived from other considerations. It is reasonable to proceed from this point of view providing one realizes what is happening. And again, what happens is that the high visibility problems surface and become the crying targets for a "where" oriented community program.

In my experience in a mental health center with a catchment area, "where" approach, the above proved accurate. Although our group initially programmed for general psychiatric disorders, we felt the pull towards the high visibility problems of juvenile crime, unemployment, alcoholism, and addiction, geriatrics and mental retardation, soon after we were operational. It led some to wish we had planned originally for these high visibility problems and it led others to frustration since few of these visibility problems are "attractive" or "responsive" to the psychiatric and para-psychiatric professions. So despite an earlier general orientation, the consequence of a "where" approach may shift the focus of attention elsewhere.

A collateral effect of this horizontal concept of community is to place a pseudo-sociologic aura to one's

7. Pasamanick, B., Scarpitti, F.R., Dinitz, S.: *Schizophrenics in the Community,* New York: Appleton-Century-Crofts, 1967.
8. Srole, L., Langer, T.S., Michael, S.T., Opler, M.K., Rennie, T.A.: *Mental Health In the Metropolis,* New York: McGraw-Hill, 1962.

efforts. This may be an exciting prospect initially as one becomes imbued with the sense of innovation and the illusion of being an instrument of social change. However, illusion it is, because entrance to the social institutions which create and devour the social condition requires skills, power, and time beyond the resources of the mental health center as a collective force or the psychiatrist as a well-meaning individual. The problem is that an aura does exist and it takes time before this aura is recognized for what it is. During the interim, staff and program may easily be pulled down the road to its inevitable disillusioning dead-end.

WHEN: Community as epiphenomenon

One of the alternate ways to consider the concept of community is to place it into a dimension of time. We have all been aware, at one time or another, of a sense of community which comes and then goes. People commonly band together to accomplish certain discrete goals and then disband. Organizations often prove to be "when" communities as they bring people together in common pursuit over a period of time. If we wished to look back, with a reverent historical purview, to the feudal gemeinschaft communities, we would still note the dissolution of that communal form over time.

Time, of course, changes all things or more correctly, all things change in time. The great leveler of human grandiosity, history, has been able to chronicle, with predictable certainty, the demise of all sorts of social organizations.[9] Civilizations and families alike are modified or terminated. But too great a preoccupation with the dimension of time becomes distressing and discouraging. After all, we must acknowledge our own temporal finiteness and the even

9. In their historical-philosophic volume, *The Lessons of History* (New York: Simon and Schuster, 1968) Will and Ariel Durant masterfully summarize the endless growth and decay of civilization as seen in the broad sweep of history.

greater temporal finiteness of our work. To feel that one's work must endure forever or to fear that one's work will be washed away immediately is to be equally absurd at either pole.

The hard core reality of the temporal dilemma is that it is very difficult to correctly estimate (*a*) if the phenomenon we are observing is an artifact of the time or a durable reality and (*b*) if our response to the phenomenon is appropriate to its duration. Is it a short range solution to a long range problem or conversely a long range solution to a short range problem? The dilemma is more often than not worked out in retrospect.

When time is applied to concepts of community, it brings to them an element of uncertainty which should humble the community expert. Most so-called communities are so time bound that they come and go like evanescent clouds. The conditions which create a community are themselves so fragile that community itself is more correctly an epiphenomenon than a primary reality in its own right. This concept of community as epiphenomenon is exceedingly important for anyone who is working in "community oriented" work. An epiphenomenon is a phenomenon which occurs as a result of pre-existing phenomena or set of conditions. An epiphenomenon is nothing unless the pre-existing events occur. And likewise a community, in its "when" sense, does not exist unless certain conditions exist.[10]

These necessary conditions would seem quite important to recognize, yet it is extraordinary to witness the degree to which they are ignored by "community oriented" workers. There is probably no greater cohesive force by which people come together into an epiphenomenon community, than that of oppression. The history of the Jews

10. Epiphenomenon, simply defined, is a secondary phenomenon accompanying another and caused by it. There is, for example, a theory of mind called epiphenomenalism which states that mental processes are epiphenomena of brain processes.

and now the Black experience in this country are graphic documentation of this fact. To take away the oppression is to take away much of the binding power of the community. To take away the oppression is to dissolve the epiphenomenon.

Working classes after the Industrial Revolution learned the lesson well and the organized labor movement in this country was the epiphenomenon of that capitalistic oppression. Even today, unions are maintained as organizations only as well as management is able to play the role of potential oppressors, or to be placed in that role by union leaders.

Oppression is only one of two necessary conditions for the epiphenomenal community. The second is leadership. That sense of shared values, common goals and kinship which is community must be articulated and transmitted to those persons who are to comprise the community. An oppressed people remain fragmented and isolated as long as no one stands to call them together, point out their common plight, articulate their frustration and present a plan for joint effort. Community implies unity and unity implies the condensation of many voices to one or few. Given the two necessary conditions, oppression and leadership, a community is born; take either of them away and the epiphenomenon vanishes.

A predictable objection arises here. Is it not so that there are examples of communities which persist without these two pre-conditions? Is not the family such a community? Again we must return to the distinction made earlier between gemeinschaft and gesellschaft communities. The gemeinschaft community exists only in rare instances outside family life. The traditions and way of life which nourished and sustained the gemeinschaft community are gone. And so we see as the prevalent form the gesellschaft community. It is my contention that there are episodic variations in the usual gesellschaft model which tend to take on the characteristics of the gemeinschaft community and that these variations occur as a result of two major conditions coming together. The resulting "sense" of community lasts only as long as these conditions and so the "gemeinschaft" community is not a durable gemeinschaft at all but rather a fragile state which we can term an epiphenomenon.

There are several implications of this perspective for community psychiatry. Those community mental health programs which have developed in suburban or affluent areas are characteristically oriented towards the provision of services to individuals or families. Their community orientation is primarily geographic and a function of fixing responsibility for various services. They have inadvertently but accurately perceived the lack of gemeinschaft. On the other hand those community mental health programs that have developed in urban centers, with a predominantly Black and oppressed constituency, have noted a sense of community and have tried in myriad ways to relate to that sense of community. It is here that the confusion is generated.

If a mental health center assumes that the community is bound together in an historical and romantic way and makes overtures for joint responsibilities, it will soon enough discover that the community will act and respond "as community" only in those issues directly related to oppression or related to the roles and prerogatives of their leaders. It will not receive a sustained community input on those more pedestrian issues that have to do with the delivery of psychiatric services. If the psychiatric services can somehow be brought into the oppression equation, then interest may exist but it will be short-lived. Again I must clarify this statement. Community interest—that is, the *representative* sentiment of a large group of persons, expressed by responsible leadership—can be sustained only in those areas directly related to their binding power as a community, *i.e.* the binding power of oppression and leadership. The interest in a mental health program can be generated in isolated "community" individuals who for one reason or another are interested in mental health matters, but do *not* assume that these interested individuals can represent a community in matters other than those related to their oppression. Even in the latter area representative views are difficult to identify.

The confusion is brought into stark relief when the community mental health center seeks to "find" its community. "Who speaks for the community?" is the plaintive cry. The answer of course is that there is no community out there, as there is no community out in the suburbs unless you are interested in getting to the epiphenomenal community, which is there for reasons already noted. In that case, the response is a relatively predictable one—and it is inexorably linked to issues of great social import. That community voice will speak to the mental health center about oppression and demand that the center take a role in their struggle. Many centers have and will attempt to get into that struggle. They are then epiphenomenal centers which will ultimately depend for their existence on the maintenance of an oppressed community.

If a center "turns its back to the community" and selects out those residents of the area interested in the center's conception of mental health services, it then runs the high risk of being identified as not truly a "community" mental health center.

HOW: Community as instrument

If the foregoing concept of epiphenomenal community is plausible, then what remains to be discussed is the functional role of that tentative community. If there are urban communities, marked by oppression and secondary communal "togetherness," then *how* do they operate in their common goals? What is the basis of their instrumental effectiveness? Although there are many ways to address these questions, I shall select the following approach because it captures the reality of today's urban life.

The ultimate instrumental force with which a "community" may attempt to impose its collective will is that of confrontation. After all, there would be no "community" had there not first been a condition of oppression and hence a state of imminent conflict. The very creative force responsible for the emergence of community is itself a real or imagined threat and so the counter force is its putative equal, counterthreat.

The point of this is to identify the fundamental force which, on the one hand serves as the community's power and, on the other, as a reinforcement of its sense of being an oppressed victim and hence a reinforcement of its sense of community. This force of confrontation must be analyzed into its various forms and a would-be provider of "community mental health services" must accurately perceive its proper relation vis-a-vis these forms of confrontation.

A community has at least four levels of confrontation that it can mobilize: (1) as physical force; (2) as anti-participant; (3) as franchiser; (4) as consumer.

Physical force

This type of confrontation leaves little to the imagination and essentially is a call to violent opposition. It has become a common device in today's urban brinkmanship and is characterized by a burst from threat to action. It should be clear that the relationship of a mental health center to its "community" cannot be fashioned after this type of functional community role.[11]

11. The "take-over" approach, wherein "community" persons literally force institutional personnel out of offices etc., and then proceed to effectively close down the operation of the institution, is an example of the physical force approach. As a technique for a community to impose its collective will upon an institution, it is the most dramatic. When applied to a fragile institution, like a community mental health center, it promotes confusion and dismemberment.

Anti-participant

A community may view an institution as so contrary to its needs that it must take a vocal stand in opposition to its existence. One can imagine the mental health center whose real or imagined program is thought to be a further instrument of societal oppression. With that provocation a community could urge that no one participate as patient or employee or in support of the center. Again, this hostile relationship can hardly serve as a model for center-community interaction. It is a fact, however, that many centers are being described as instruments of social oppression and militant opposition has developed in many instances. But again let us draw out the important distinction. Although there may be articulate and militant opponents to a program, it is a non-sequitur to ascribe this opposition to the ubiquitous "community." Truly anti-participant reaction from "the community," *i.e.* a broad level, grass-roots opposition, could develop only if a center could (*a*) capture the attention of the entire community, (*b*) behave in a blatantly oppressive fashion so as to generate their cohesive opposition, and/or (*c*) through distorted charges of great magnitude, be incorrectly perceived as oppressor. These are extremely unlikely conditions and so also is a truly anti-participatory response from the community.

Franchiser

A community takes on a special relationship with a center if it is in the position of franchiser. This suggests ultimate sponsorship by the community, with consequent control (or "power" in today's vocabulary) of program, personnel and funds. On the face of it this would seem an ideal way for a community to "confront" an institution which attempts to provide it service.[12] However, the magic of the word covers the underlying absurdity. A commu-

12. Smith, M.B., Hobbs, N.: *The Community and the Community Mental Health Center,* Washington, D.C.: American Psychological Association, 1966.

nity, in its true sense, does not organize itself in such a way so as to provide an authoritative control over an institution.[13] It will not yield a "representative" body with the abiding interest and competence to "control" so idiosyncratic an institution as a mental health center. To be sure, isolated individuals from here and there, for this reason or that, will rise "on behalf of the community" but there is little reason to expect in them the mandate or wisdom of the people for whom they wish to speak. It very quickly becomes an argument based on the visceral feeling . . . a little community is better than none at all isn't it?

Let us assume however that a community has developed its own internal system of representative voice and action. There are communities of this type. Here, I am not referring to the usual governmental structures which in their own way are "representative," but rather refer to area organizations (such as in the Woodlawn area of Chicago).[14] Such organizations have a way of maintaining their identity for functions far removed from their original intent. An organization formed to deal with housing or education could conceivably provide the sponsorship of a mental health center but to suppose that it is a "community" vehicle for control, support and responsibility may or may not follow. If the level of communication and mutual trust between the people of the community and the representative organization is consistent and durable, then it may well be an ideal franchiser of mental health services. It

13. The closest society has come to success in exerting truly collective will over its institutions is the republic form of government. Through the processes of nomination and election, the masses have delegated certain decision making rights to others. We are all aware of the enormous problems in this orientation, with political expediency, inevitable priority conflicts and parochialism. Self-appointed "representatives" constantly muddy the already murky waters.

14. Kellam, S.G., and Schiff, S.K., The Woodlawn Mental Health Center, *Soc. Sci. Rev.* 40:255, 1966.

would be naive, however, to hope to create a new community organization concurrently with a new mental health center. Both require enormous amounts of dedication, sophistication and organizational skill. To have two mutually dependent institutions go through their separate and idiosyncratic processes together is to invite their mutual dissolution.

Consumer

The ultimate power of a community is that inherent in those persons who, by common need, accept or reject the role of service consumer. If the goal of an institution, like a mental health center, is to provide a service, then there can be no greater control than that which operates in the decision of a consumer to use or not use the service. To be able to extend this "power" to "the community" necessitates a relatively free market atmosphere. It means the provision of alternative services and the right of patients to choose that service which more closely meets *their* idiosyncratic need.[15] To close the options by creating catchment area boundaries is to imprison the people of that area and to insure their dependence on what could be an arbitrary mental health program whether by professional design or by design of those "professional" community representatives who speak with neither mandate nor clear vision.

The dilemma becomes clearer, however, when we fully appreciate the impasse. Given a catchment area exclusivity, we find a community voice impossible or improbable in each of the four functional strategies open to it. This leaves us with a peculiar conclusion: A community mental health center is neither of the community, by the community, nor for the community.

Given the reality of today's catchment area approach,

15. Adam Smith's view of economic equilibrium leaned heavily on the belief that the need-demand vs. supply principle in an open market economy would ultimately work to the benefit of both the consumer and the supplier.

with the consequent closed market for the consumer, the only viable functional role left for "the community" is as franchiser. As already noted, however, this will only be possible in rare instances. Again, at the risk of being redundant, let us restate that the concept of community in the foregoing refers to the evanescent gemeinschaft still to be found in oppressed populations. It refers to their collective and therefore representative needs and demands and *not* to the interpreted needs and demands of a pseudocommunity as articulated by self-appointed "representatives."

COMMUNITY CONTROL: Grassroots and Weeds

Community mental health centers face the same dilemma in relating to community as do all other service-oriented institutions. They are considerably more at risk because of connotations of terms like mental illness and mental health. Having been born into times of accelerated change they can hardly succeed in forging a self-identity. People are now "seeing" irrelevance in all or most institutions and so the wish or demand for institutional change runs rampant. "If they can't make their institution more relevant we will!" So goes the cry from the people . . . or at least some of the people. The "they" are usually thought of as alien, hostile and malevolent while the "we" are dedicated, altruistic and intrinsically instrumental. In today's heightened atmosphere of confrontation, the way to resolve a problem is to "confront" it.

The balance to the above is that many institutions are in fact unable to meet increased demands. The demands are now quantitatively and qualitatively more complex. The charge of irrelevance becomes an issue and a fact as long as the "demands" are not carefully defined and as long as priorities within institutions are not set. An institution that says to a community, "we shall attack mental illness" or "we shall promote mental health" is simply setting itself up for the rejoinder "you are irrelevant."

And so the issue of community influence, whether as the franchiser or as consumer is integrally linked to the issue of program goals. Someone has to decide what they shall be. A community will never succeed in imposing its goals on a center that is unwilling. And a center will never succeed in imposing its goals on a community if there are no consumers. The commonplace "battle for control" is an exercise in futility for both combatants.

A starting point is imperative. Let us start at the community end. If the foregoing has any merit we can anticipate two relevant community roles: (1) as franchiser and (2) as consumer. Either of these are possible but their possibility depends on the extant nature of the particular community in question. As I have indicated, a franchising community necessitates an existing "representative" body. The "incorporation" of interested community persons is an exercise in illusion. The incorporated body is as much a *special interest group* as any institution. Their special interest will emerge from their own narrow perspectives. To be willing to relate to such a franchising group is no different than relating to any institutional franchiser. To relate to a true community franchiser is desirable but difficult to attain.

What seems a rational premise is that the search for the "community" be abandoned. A search for the grail would be as rewarding. What then should a mental health center set about to do vis-a-vis its "community?" Contrary to the romantic readiness to do the community will, a mental health center must know, in advance, what it is it can do and wishes to do. Armed with this sense of identity and purpose it can turn to "its community" and identify itself. As part of its process of deciding what it is and what it can and wishes to do, it must also decide to what degree it wishes to balance its internal decision making processes by the inclusion of persons *identifiable* as (*a*) area residents; (*b*) vitally interested in the work of the center; (*c*) with the ability to conceptualize the types of problems and types of solutions involved; (*d*) with a willingness to *participate* and an ability to disagree as well as agree. This is "organizational sensitization," *i.e.* the conscious internal process of keeping an organization open to the life style and "needs" of its potential consumers. This is a process that should be initiated from within the Center. It cannot easily be imposed from without because that breeds organizational coercion and not sensitization. If a center's leadership does not choose to support and welcome the voices of its potential consumers then it simply will not have a sensitized organization. One may wish it to be otherwise but the difference between rhetoric and performance lies within those who must perform. This is nowhere more true than in the highly personalized and complex task of intervening in human behavior. As long as an organization can maintain an internal system of self-regulation so as to constantly focus and re-focus on its task, it will remain viable. This internal system of self-regulation will not work well unless it is truly internalized, *i.e.* unless there are multilevel consumer-oriented inputs.[16] The dependence on external inputs, such as with the common use of an advisory board structure, quickly degenerates into a pro forma relationship if there is no internal system of consumer influence.

Some centers have been able to maintain organizational sensitization by carefully seeing to it that area residents who meet the aforementioned criteria are hired for "meaningful" jobs within the center. The indigenous worker trend may be more important because of its influence as an agent of organizational sensitization than for its more explicit manpower resource role. If this is working well

16. No consumer-oriented institution can survive unless it pays attention to its market. The market research department, within consumer-oriented industry, is a fundamental system which keeps organizational goals relevant to consumer needs. An analogic system within community mental health centers is critical.

then good balance can come from an adivsory board structure, providing the advisors and the internal staff have
open communication with each other.

The point to all of this is to de-mythologize the term
community and re-focus the issue around organizational
sensitization. Simply stated this means the awareness of an
organization of the multiple problems, some subtle and
some not, related to doing its task. It implies neither a
predetermined task nor one arrived at by representative
election. Presumably there are some tasks for which persons in the mental health professions are particularly
suited and some for which they are not. Once those tasks
are made clear and decided on as organizational goals,
then, and only then, should an organization turn to its
potential consumer for help in maintaining its awareness to
the problems in reaching its goals. If those goals are not
the ultimate goals of a "community" (presuming those
could be discovered), then it will simply become a service
institution for a population group, with a priority (or
"relevance") less than ultimate. It means being willing to
see oneself as less than the savior institution and being
willing to say to "community" voices that the mental
health center is not the grand instrument of social renovation.

ISSUE OF BLACK AND WHITE

This dilemma about community must be placed into
perspective, especially with respect to its racial implications. The popularization of the concept of community is
a corollary to the entire social awareness reaction of the
last decade.[17] One of the fundamental catalysts of this
social consciousness has been and continues to be the
Negro struggle for equality. The tragic dimensions of this

17. In Durant (op. cit. 1968), one can appreciate the historical
    tendency for an alternation between concern for the individual
    and concern for society.

social revolution dwarf other processes involved in institutional renovation. Nearly every institution is caught up in its own attempt at renewal but the contagion and drama of the Negro plight have attached themselves to these various institutions. Their own future course now becomes enmeshed in the working out of the Black identity process.

It is conceivable that because community psychiatry has come into vogue in the wake of the Black revolution, its own identity and working through will be confounded by the vagaries of the more historically profound movement. There is a double-edged sword here. On the one hand, the moral impetus of the Black revolution has imbued the community psychiatry movement with an aura of moral righteousness and therefore its personnel has been enthusiastic and committed. On the other hand it has created a whole series of illusory goals, abstractly related to sacred concepts of mental health, and therefore it may have sealed its own ultimate frustration. Highly committed persons in an inevitably frustrating task . . . therein lies the potential tragic element.

The movements are distinct and separate. One, the Black revolution, is profound and touches the total fabric of our social structure. The other, the community psychiatry movement, is a moment in time, a transition stage between a narrow view of care to the mentally ill and a broader view with yet uncertain borders. Each has its own goals and processes. To begin to apply the jargon of mental health, developed to understand the individual, to institutions, communities and value systems, is to invite the collective wrath of those whose expectations will have been raised beyond our capacity.

There are so many red herrings with racial implications in the community psychiatry movement, that it is common to see the staff of a large urban mental health center devour itself as it seeks some new guilt reducing strategy. The amount of effort turned towards a therapeutic community approach becomes enormous. The irony, however, is that the object of this therapeutic preoccupation is the center staff *itself* and not those persons for whom presumably the center exists. To ignore the reality of racial bias and its effects on the personnel of a center would be naive but preoccupation with organizational cleansing is a trap as self-limiting as any.

chapter 2

PLANNING AND DEVELOPMENT:

An Arrow Into the Wind

DEFINING MENTAL HEALTH

It is a presumption of leadership that futuristic ideas can be brought to reality by a plan of action. Alfred North Whitehead condemned ideas, regardless of their brilliance, if they were not followed by action.[1] Action in the absence of design, without the guidance of plan, is generally considered futile and inefficient. And yet, the process of planning is, more often than we care to admit, a flight into illusion. To plan effectively is to presume control of all or most of the variables which play a role. No planner is ever in control of all the variables and he is less in control when the end product of his planning, the idea itself, is vague and ill-defined. The planner of a program for "mental health" is in real trouble right from the begin-

1. Whitehead, A.N.: *Science and the Modern World,* New York: The Macmillan Co., 1925.

ning. There are no generally acceptable definitions of "mental health," nor are there any for "mental illness."

A state of conceptual ambiguity has been generated by the recent turning of attention towards social and community psychiatry. The tendency to suspend the conceptual restrictions imposed by our archaic nomenclature and the immersion of psychiatrists into socio-cultural "catchment areas" have broadened perspectives but also upset the tenuous reassurances afforded by our prior "understanding" of the unifying concept, "mental illness" and its equally reassuring opposite, "mental health." How are socio-cultural "problems" to be distinguished from psychiatric "illness?" Is juvenile delinquency a manifestation of social disorder or mental disorder? What are the criteria for "mental illness?"

Inherent in the confusion is the compartmental narrowness and consequent polarization of all of those academic disciplines concerned with understanding behavior. This intra-disciplinary allegiance, with the associated development of intra-disciplinary data, language and generalization has predictably generated the tunnel vision answers of Freud as well as of Durkheim.[2] Our movement toward "psychosocial" concern is nothing more than expanded tunnel vision. We now choose to attend to another level while yet ignoring others. It is because of the enormous complexity of data "within" a discipline like sociology that we hesitate to go beyond it. It is because of our data-consciousness that we find ourselves overwhelmed by individual particles of information and unable to move to

2. When looked at through a telescope, generalizing as best one can from their many contributions, one can discern a fundamental divergence between Freud and Durkheim. Freud was ultimately led to attributing human behavior to forces residing within the individual. His was a determinism of psychologic pre-eminence. Durkheim, on the other hand, was fundamentally committed to the proposition that human behavior was determined primarily by forces outside of the individual. His was a determinism of socio-cultural pre-eminence.

the broader levels of generalization. Being much less resourceful than the digital computer, we are content to stay within a workable discipline with its more limited range of data, variation and language.

It is this pragmatic conservatism that has allowed us to consider mental disorder and social disorder as dichotomous or mutually exclusive rather than continuous. And yet there is validity in choosing to organize certain kinds of data into a discipline and to exclude other data. To do otherwise would be the supreme tautology. Boulding stated it well: "This is General Systems Theory. It does not seek, of course, to establish a single, self-contained general theory of practically everything which will replace all the special theories of particular disciplines. Such a theory would be almost without content, for we always pay for generality by sacrificing content, and all we can say about practically everything is almost nothing. Somewhere, however, between the specific that has no meaning and the general that has no content there must be, for each purpose and at each level of abstraction, an optimum degree of generality."[3]

The issue is most painful when planned action or intervention is expected to come from an understanding of the data of a discipline. If the data which order intervention can be found within one discipline, then the relationship between the agent of intervention (the art) and the discipline (the science) is mutually creative. This is the case in the relationship between the art of surgery and the "sciences" of anatomy and physiology. This is not the case with the art of psychiatry and its complementary science. In a very real sense the "science" or "sciences" that could provide the resource for psychiatry have never been adequately identified. We abstractly refer to the "behavioral sciences" but do not meaningfully relate to them. In so far as psychiatry has been an "applied psychology," it has

3. Boulding, K.E., General Systems Theory—the Skeleton of Science, *Management Science*, 2 (1956), 197—208.

presumed certain limits; but its medical and biologic origins, as well as its "socio-cultural" concerns, are broader in implication and application than can be subsumed by any extant psychology.

Psychiatry's implicit concern with behavior places it foresquare in inter-relation with all scientific disciplines which are concerned with behavior. Human behavior then and not "mental illness" is the principal object of study. The art may be intervention into selected behaviors ("mental illness?") but this presumes an articulated understanding of "ordered" as well as "disordered" behavior whether on the level of validated law or theoretical model.

As Jahoda has pointed out, the concepts of mental health and mental illness are extraordinarily ambiguous.[4] The general category "health" and its antithesis, "disease," which provide the sine qua non of medical nomenclature, can give only orienting help.

Another way of saying all of this is that we must be conceptually clear as to what the object of our planning is to be and that it must be neither too broad so as to "include everything" nor too restrictive so as to exclude what is meaningful. But having led the reader to a humble beginning is to also lead the planner to a tenuous starting point.

The legislative guidelines for the development of Community Mental Health Centers[5/6] show that the definition of mental health or mental illness has escaped the legislators as well. What are mandated are the minimum service structures (*i.e.* in-patient care, out-patient care, partial hospitalization, emergency service, consultation and education, etc.).

And so the planner is immediately seduced into a dread-

4. Jahoda, M.: *Current Concepts of Positive Mental Health,* New York: Basic Books, Inc., 1958.
5. Joint Commission On Mental Illness and Health: *Action For Mental Health,* New York: Basic Books, 1961.
6. Congress of the United States: Mental Retardation Facilities and Community Mental Health Centers Act of 1963. Public Law 88-164.

ful short-cut. He plans for the means without identifying the ends. Five well-staffed, well-oiled and administratively sound structures do *not* mental health make. To add to the confusion, a key concept is eased in, clothed in the stuff of Americana, the flag and glory—the concept of community. This is no more easily defined than is mental health and so when laid end to end—community mental health—one can find much to confuse.[7]

This now leads logically, or so it now seems, to a fundamental starting point. *Define that for which you are to plan.* Don't become enthralled with the ultimate definition, a definition to withstand the sands of time, a definition for all men, a definition which will dazzle the eye and boggle the mind. This is not to say that any old definition will do, but certainly between the sublime ("the treatment of psychosis") and the ridiculous ("the removal of sociocultural inequity") there are many ideologically sound definitions that are operationally feasible.

It is more than important to indicate clearly that there is NO ONE ideal definition. The one which is *selected* may be more or less feasible. But the important thing is that a choice is made while acknowledging that no choice is perfect. "This will be what we mean when we say mental illness." The corollary then is "that will *not* be what we mean when we say mental illness."

To one who has not yet stepped into the quivering world of community psychiatry the rationality of the above may seem so inevitable that he questions this as a blinding glimpse of the obvious. However, the merits of

7. One of the prices we pay for a democratic form of government is the inevitable frustration of planning. Strong and durable central governments of a more oligarchic type insure control over more variables (*i.e.* less freedom) and therefore insure a more reasonable expectation of carrying through with plans. It is interesting to note that within the general context of a democratic liberal governmental establishment, the most efficient of our institutions are those in the private industrial sector, with strong, undemocratic, centralized controls.

such an approach become apparent in the inevitable tensions and conflicts which come in time as new true believers see their version of the ultimate definition. Unless one has gone through the painstaking process of selection, the introduction of new and highly charged alternative goals can undermine years of effort.

The counter-arguments to early definition of mental health goals usually rest on other sacrosanct concepts of the community psychiatry movement. Innovation is one of these concepts. It becomes somehow axiomatic that to define goals is to become instantly rigid, immensely authoritarian, anti-participatory and worst of all—traditional. Although one can be committed to innovation, exploration, participation, and egalitarianism, these are not mutually exclusive with working towards ends. If certain ends are not to your liking, then you are free to get off the trolley and go elsewhere. But at least you will know that this trolley has a destination.

Concepts of innovation and its many bed-fellows are operational and not necessarily addressed to goals. Innovation should be applied to *ways* of getting to the end-point. The end-point itself is not an innovative construct. If it is, then throw it out, unless you are prepared to build on a very tentative foundation.

INNOVATION: throwing the bath water out with the baby

One of the sacred words in the new psychiatry is innovation. It is a cleansing word because it suggests an out with the old and in with the new mentality. It is fresh, creative, experimental, free and good. It is energized with goodwill, commitment and ingenuity. It is anti-establishment, anti-tradition, anti-failure and anti-stuffiness. It is optimistic, egalitarian, and benevolent. In a word, it is sacred.

Granting the obvious declarations that things change and times change, and needs change, it follows that the processes at work within change are important. New ideas are important as are new methods. Without the new and the change that gets us there, progress would end. But this string of obvious truth does not include an inevitable joyous celebration for all innovation. Most of it is junk. Most of it is borne in the expanded ego of its creator. Most of it leans heavily on assumptions crammed full with personal values. Most of it takes up valuable time, effort and money and gives its creators a brief moment onstage with the spotlight glaring. Again, most of it is junk.

Tradition and How it Happened

How is it that you are a biped with erect posture, not only knowing but also knowing that you know? You share these unique features with all of humankind and so are not really that unique. The sameness of humans is a function of evolutionary success. This form, this adaptive structure, does well enough to reproduce its kind and wage life with the environment. Evolution discarded many innovations before settling on traditional old you.

The moral could be: "don't knock what works!" but it could also be: "what works survives!" There is more than a little wisdom in the latter aphorism. Fortunately there seems to be a built-in mechanism in our collective common sense which is eminently practical. Theories, ideas, inspirations and proposals all eventually are tested by economic pragmatism. Only a few survive; the rest are accorded some homage in journals, history books or adolescent cults. The confusing fact, however, is that the time lag between the idea and its ultimate testing can be quite long. Society seems quite hospitable to anyone's idea, giving it a honeymoon for a variable length of time. But eventually it gets squeezed by other ideas and other priorities. Eventually it has to work or die. While waiting to find out, however, some men ride their innovative illusion for quite a while. Society is naive in the short run but critical and wise in the long run.

The concept of tradition has a meaning that should be made explicit. Webster's says, "the handing down of information, beliefs and customs by word of mouth or by example from one generation to another without written instruction." Tradition therefore is a part of culture. It is not something easily dismissed, forgotten or changed. But neither is there any inherent sense of eternity about tradition. It can and does change but the point here is that it is durable and somewhat procrustean in that it often disregards individual differences or special circumstances. And there is the irritant. We have been increasingly sensitive to individual differences and in fact it is the special sign of the psychiatrist that he is constantly alert to individual differences. Tradition is an accumulation of generalizations. It is never easily applicable to the individual. It is therefore in constant jeopardy when face to face with the advocates of the individual.

Problem solving, whether it be of a psychiatric sort or some other behavioral kind, is extraordinarily difficult. It is difficult because the number of variables in any behavioral segment is enormous. No one interventional technique can address itself to all of the essential variables and so the pragmatic problem solver goes to great lengths to restrict the focus of his intervention. He carefully defines "the" problem from among the many that can be controlled in their essential variables. The idealistic problem solver will recognize the futility of established techniques in broad-based problems. He will reject them as "irrelevant" and proceed to construct an innovation designed to have impact on the broader problem. In some ways it is like choosing between a cannon aimed at an insect (pragmatist) and a pea-shooter aimed at an elephant (idealist).

There is a built-in illusion in either example. The pragmatist must act "as if" the focus of his intervention exists in pure culture, *i.e.* unconnected to the rest of the "patient's" life circumstances. This illusion is difficult to maintain. One of the most frequent devices used by the pragmatic problem solver, which serves to maintain the illusion, is a preoccupation with technique. He will be very sensitive to the "correct" way to interpret the patient's comments or the "correct" way to respond to those comments, or the "correct" amount of involvement he should pursue. He will control his intervention and limit it with correctness as his guide.

The idealistic problem solver suffers from the illusion of contagious causality. He "sees" the connections between problems. The poverty is connected to the impulses, the alcoholism is connected to oppression, the depression is connected to overcrowding. This global interconnectedness (which is quite valid in its own right) is then displaced to treatment strategy. To intervene at the more general levels (*e.g.* oppression or overcrowding) is felt to be connected to results at the specific levels (*e.g.* alcoholism or depression). The device used to maintain this illusion is a surrender of specific individually oriented goals for the more general goals. It comes out sounding: "If we can influence oppression, poverty and overcrowding, then there will be less depression and alcoholism." Even if one wishes to grant the correctness of this approach, the net effect is to ignore the individual for the sake of the general *without* strategy, expertise, resources or mandate. He is the innovator par excellence.

The point is that innovation should spring from tradition. It should maintain a connection with tradition if only to point out its divergence from that tradition. An innovation that springs up de novo, as a totally new approach (if that is really possible), has maybe a 5% chance of surviving over the long haul. If one likes those odds (and smells a short cut to the Nobel prize) one might persist. But a wise administrator would insist that the more radical the innovation (*i.e.* the further from traditional wisdom) the more restricted to pilot status that innovation should be kept.

Psychiatry labors under the strain and support of traditions but they are not "psychiatric traditions." It is commonplace to hear the innovative-minded mental health professional deplore the use of traditional psychiatric methods. This suggests that there is a culture or ethos within psychiatry that dictates the methods used. This "tradition" is seen as part of the "medical model" where a physician cares for a patient in a one-to-one service oriented encounter. But the "traditional" psychiatric method and its bedfellow, the "medical model" are not traditional. They are not handed down from generation to generation, with assumptive value attached. They are not culturally transmitted methods. The medical model is based on very practical reality. Every state of equilibrium or disequilibrium has *at least* two interactants. If a sick person wishes to be helped, he must be related to by at least one other person who can help. There are numerous beneficial results which can be afforded a patient by bringing him into a medical relationship with a doctor. That level of interaction, *i.e.* the medical model, is valid and appropriate for certain levels of intervention. There is nothing traditional about it. It is practical, successful and necessary for certain results. To say that there are other desirable results which cannot be accomplished through the medical model is an insight as profound as saying that the climate in New York is different than it is in Florida. Neither Florida nor New York have "traditional" climates. Their climates are simply different. And so too the psychiatric method (if by that one conjures up a one-to-one encounter) is simply different than another variation, whatever it might be. When one appreciates the enormous variations within the medical model (*i.e.* within the one-to-one encounter), it is hard to understand how they can be lumped together in so cavalier a fashion.

One good test of the innovator's value is to note the degree to which he feels obliged to attack other methods. If he must climb on the corpse of a pre-existing method and beat his chest, then he is probably part of another new religion. If an innovator can pass up the opportunity to destroy what already exists, it may indicate that he is more interested in pursuing truth than in erecting monuments. There are an enormous variety of problems of all sorts and at all levels of human organization. They are going to require an enormous variety of "treatment" approaches from the medical model to all kinds of others. To righteously proclaim that the medical model does not work for the problem of rats in the kitchen, is to perpetuate the myth that medicine should be able, not only to understand all of the problems that ultimately impinge on human health, but also be the direct change agent for all of these problems. That is to make of medicine the biggest daddy of them all.

Basic Elements

There are some basic elements or ' guidelines which should help in keeping the concept of innovation within the realm of reason. These elements will be developed from the peculiar perspective of community psychiatry and the structure of the mental health center. First of all innovation must be *in the service of the goals* which order a mental health center. An innovation which leads to a result inconsistent with center goals should not be entertained regardless of the nobility of the innovative goal. This is a chronic problem in the mental health center that includes changes in the social order in its goals. If those changes are not explicitly stated in the statement of goals then widely divergent programs can spring up. At this stage of development, mental health centers can hardly afford to be conglomerates.

Innovations should not be entertained until their creators have *explicitly searched history and the literature* to note the progenitors or historical precedents of their innovation. This should dispel the de novo mystique which accompanies many old ideas in new trappings. Community psychiatry programs in America generally fail to recognize their historical legacy from Beers, Meyer, and other early century advocates of social awareness. They fail to capitalize on the experiences of France, England and the Scandinavian countries, which have a long tradition of social medicine. They fail to recognize the great body of information available in the social sciences and the great number of myths these sciences have already laid to rest.

Innovations should not be entertained unless they are *expressed in articulate and measurable concepts.* The alternative to this is to continue capitalizing on the longevity of illusion. If it can neither be proven valuable nor worthless, then an innovative program joins the ever-growing mass of clutter. It distracts people from the real task of finding something that works and betrays those who need something that works.

Innovations should not be entertained until they are *expressed in clear operational terms.* If the innovation is attractive by virtue of the result it hopes to achieve, then it should also be attractive by virtue of its operational uniqueness and advantage. How this operation is to proceed, *i.e.* who does what to whom, when and why, is of critical importance. It may be too much to expect a program to be spelled out in great detail from beginning to end before it is undertaken; but it is not too much to ask that the creator of the innovation be aware of where and how he would *like* to see his program go.[8]

Staff Stability

We must accept at the start that not all men are as wise as we. How else could it be, in view of the resistance of some to our brilliant plans? The beauty for an artist is that he can create alone. He must master the instruments and techniques of his art but then he is free to do what he wishes. But when two or more people come together, the artist in each of them comes out, and resents the other. Egalitarian collaboration is a disguised exercise in sophisticated competition. How to win without blood is the game.

8. The explicit rules of decision making within an organization are its by-laws. No organization can continue for long unless it has explicity stated by-laws.

Innovative programs have an interesting effect on this process of collaborative competition. The important ingredient at the outset is salesmanship. Since the product is basically untested, the creator of the idea has to sell his idea over and over again. Presuming he has been successful enough to get to a point where he has people hired to work on a project, he now faces the task of selling his staff on his ideas. If he is good at this (a general rule: an innovator is always a better salesman than he is a producer of goods) then his staff will be imbued with a high level of motivation. It is invariably exciting to be involved in something new. Discovery and surprise are potent motivators. This flush of excitement brings out an unusual (and short-lived) quantity of self-sacrifice and subservience. The staff of an innovative program will glory in their exclusivity. Toleration for one another is extended and failure is "understood" as a temporary corollary to a new bold venture.[9]

What is happening during this early flush phase is that the creator of the innovation is able to draw heavily on his credit. But what is also happening is that his credit deficits are being carefully noted. If he (*i.e.* the innovative program) doesn't eventually pay off, the creditors will howl in rage. By creditors here I am referring to all those staff persons who allowed themselves to become seduced into a journey towards glory. All of those naturally competitive and critical instincts will emerge with a vengeance and be turned against their leader. Partially scapegoat and partially deserved victim, the creator of a busted innovation invariably finds a job somewhere else. He feels himself living proof of the proverb that predicts no honor for a prophet in his own house.

The moral of this tale is that the creator of an innovation and the staff of the innovative program both run high risks which go beyond the simple fact of success or failure of the program. Failure often smashes hard against all

9. A further discussion of participatory and non-participatory administration follows in Chapter 4.

involved. Since failure probably attends many more innovations than does success, *caveat emptor.*

PLANNING AS MYTH AND REALITY

A mature man should have little difficulty appreciating
the self-deception inherent in the planning process. To
which of his "achievements" can he look and find the
same dimensions as in his original plan? How many efforts
have required continuous alteration of plan because of unforeseen elements? It would be truly surprising if planning
led to the point by point achievement of the plan outline.
But what is even more surprising is the degree to which
planners talk and act as if their creations are the only
way.[10/11]

Given the enormous number of variables associated with
any future event, planning, particularly in the mental
health area, is truly like the shooting of an arrow into the
wind. What can be hoped for is that the arrow will land
somewhere in the general vicinity of the target. If you
expect more than that you are doomed to frustration and
disappointment. With this realistic orientation it is possible
to anticipate an inevitable fact of organizational life:
change.

Change comes with two faces. If unanticipated it may
be ugly and disruptive. If anticipated it can be tolerated
and even creative. To some it seems contradictory to plan
for change. To plan implies a trend towards stability. To
change implies a trend towards instability. What makes
them truly contradictory is the inappropriate expectation
that becomes attached to the concept of planning. If planning is done with change as an expected and, in fact, desirable element, you will have defused a predictable, disruptive process in your program development.

10. Banfield, Edward, personal communication during meetings of
    Inter-University Forum for Educators In Community Psychi-
    atry, Chicago, October 1969.
11. Lowi, T.: *The End of Liberalism,* New York: W.W. Norton &
    Co. Inc., 1969.

OVERCOMMITMENT AND ITS CONSEQUENCES

Since mental health centers are relatively new, one would expect that their level of development would be rather primitive. The number of organizational precedents are limited and so a good deal of the task of development has had to proceed through trial and error. This method has a significant risk and many mental health centers have already been burned. The risk lies in our tendency to be overzealous and over-ambitious.[12/13] Planning in the grand scale is very American. It leads to empire building in some instances but to bankruptcy in others.

Community psychiatry and its tangible structure—the community mental health center—are both suffering from a bad case of overcommitment. Community psychiatry has committed itself to "the community" and to "mental health," without knowing what either of them are. Now the definitions are coming in from all quarters and that pulls the already overextended center into an amorphous umbrella without props. Under the federal, state and local governmental bureaucracy, its mandate shifts with every political breeze. Every angry, long-suffering, special interest group intent on pushing the cause for the treatment of mental retardation, alcoholism, juvenile crime, air pollution, poverty, or overpopulation, can now turn to the Community Mental Health Center and remind it of its "mandated duty." And the hapless mental health center, having hoisted itself on its own petard, responds by innovating itself into oblivion.

The consequence of overcommitment is agony and its cure is forthright retreat. The magic word is NO and it must be said forcefully and loudly. It would have been much easier to say if the mental health center had been the

12. Dunham, H.W.: Community Psychiatry: The Newest Therapeutic Band-Wagon, *Archives of General Psychiatry*, 12, 303–313, 1965.
13. Burrows, W.G.: Community Psychiatry—Another Bandwagon? *Canadian Psychiatric Association Journal* 14:105-14, April 1969.

child of wisdom rather than a dream born of indigestion. But now we have to work backward, setting limits where before there were boundless horizons.

The reluctant realist should keep something in mind as he faces this retreat. The same confusion and ambiguity which have been turned against him and which have expanded his mandate beyond capacity—that same confusion and ambiguity can be turned around and used on his tormenters. "Of course, we are interested in mental illness, but we do not consider overpopulation a manifestation of mental illness. A cause of mental illness? Well, that may be so but it certainly hasn't been proven to be and besides that would probably be a sociological disease. Why don't you go talk to the sociologists about it?"

"Yes commissioner, I realize that you expect me to be responsible for the 1200 patients being discharged to my catchment area next week and I will be happy to send a staff person to a task force meeting to discuss the problem. There is no task force? Well, don't you think there should be? Well, in that case you'll have to figure out what to do with those 1200 patients yourself because we are committed to mental health here and that includes the mental health of our staff."

If you don't start doing it now, a year from now some officious know-it-all will be asking you why you didn't limit your commitments . . . as you padlock the front door.

MIXING RESOURCES AND CONSTRAINTS

The two major ingredients in an analysis of program feasibility are *resources* and *constraints.* The resources are all the imaginable, in-hand, tangible things and people to help reach a goal. Constraints should be thought of in a very different dimension. Constraints relate to the time dimension. They are made specific in answering the question: how durable are these resources? In other words the concept of constraint relates to the concept of resource and *not* to the concept of goal.

With this perspective, lack of money does not qualify as a constraint. Let us assume that we have an idea based on a perceived need, *i.e.* based on a potential market. The idea (in response to the need) is that a psychiatric emergency unit should be *considered* as a goal. Before it is *established* as a goal it is necessary that sufficient resources be available. One of these resources is quite likely to be money. If there is no money, then a key resource is absent and therefore the goal is not set. The point is that a goal is not set before the resources are considered. Once a goal is set it should be presumed that there are sufficient resources to reach the goal. The problem now shifts to a consideration of all of those factors which can or will subvert the resources over *time*.

Many planners skip this last step. Having considered the idea for a goal and after having assessed the resources available, they plunge into operation. There is little, if any, thought paid to the problem of sustaining the level of resource and to anticipating future deterioration of those resources. A key example is the cataclysm which strikes a mental health center when it learns its funds may be cut. The possibility of funds being cut should have been part of the original planning and analysis of resources at the time goals were set. This constraint on resource, *i.e.* the tenuous source of finances, should have prompted contingency planning at the beginning. Now it is perfectly reasonable to expect that situations may change abruptly and undercut a resource; and it is reasonable to assert that many such changes are unpredictable. The only point we are trying to make here is that no goal should be set without prior assessment of resources and that no assessment of resources is complete until the durability of those resources is assessed. The absence of durability (*i.e.* resource viability over *time*) is a constraint.

Unless one is building a paper tower and expects it to topple with the first breeze, the foregoing issues should play a dominant role in one's planning. In the scramble of developing community mental health centers one sees a remarkable lack of appreciation of these facts. Institutions are being built for today's kicks and very often as monuments to their clever and energetic directors. A constraint is not thought of as having any meaning except at the moment of creation. And so we have creators of ideas and starters of mental health centers. What remains to be seen is whether there are many maintainers of mental health centers.

THE RELATIONSHIP BETWEEN VIRTUE AND SIZE

Whenever someone becomes involved in the character of a medical organization, one runs the risk of seeing a breakdown in what is considered to be the standard of quality. The logical next step is to attribute that breakdown to the impersonality and bigness of the organization. In the minds of many persons in the health field, from doctor to aide, is the association of bigness with badness and the association of smallness with goodness. It is often expressed as "a manageable operation," a process which is small enough to allow for control of most of the variables. The bigger the operation, the more people and the more variables and the less quality control.

This kind of thinking is no doubt responsible for the movement of many health professionals from large organizations to smaller ones, and to the ultimate small operation, the private practice. Experience certainly seems to substantiate the size vs quality equation. But within the truth of this conclusion lies a distinction that is critical. Quality is not inversely proportional to size but rather directly proportional to the control of key operational variables. If the key variables can be adequately controlled, there need be no limit to the size of an organization with maintenance of quality.

The problem of quality control is a problem of variable control and not one of size control. Of course there are more variables as the operation becomes larger but the critical control features remain the same. Once goals, methods and standards of care have been made explicit, then it becomes a management problem to keep the operations keyed to those guidelines. What frequently seems to happen is that the more sophisticated persons with management talents are clustered at the top and there is a sharp drop-off in this particular talent as one moves closer to the firing line. It is quite self-defeating to promote your talent out of the action.

But this position is little consolation to an already far-flung operation suffering from poor quality control. An important point emerges. It is far more reasonable to expand an operation a piece at a time, as each piece is carefully constructed for quality control, than it is to start on a grand scale and then work backwards to incorporate features of quality control. Personnel will resist controls when they are imposed after a period without controls. But for many mental health centers the staff is already at sea and the navigating equipment is just being developed.

It may not be easy to slow down the action but if that action is an undisciplined hodge-podge of idiosyncratic effort, with good work here, bad work there, intuition as a guideline, and uneven management—then it must be slowed down or even halted. Explicit standards must be stated and explicit controls for those standards must be established. The standards and the controls should be part and parcel of the intra-organizational reporting system so that there is an open view of where the standards are being met, missed or exceeded.

Poor quality of work is almost invariably a symptom of poor quality leadership. The size of the organization becomes a handy scapegoat but the truth of the matter is that there has not developed a clarity of expectation nor a clarity in the ways of measuring performance. When

5

people know what's expected and know that their performance can be evaluated against that expectation, then their performance will usually meet the challenge.

chapter 3

MANPOWER CONSIDERATIONS:
Doing Little with Many

We are constantly being reminded that there is not sufficient manpower for the ambitious scope of the community
mental health center movement.[1][2][3] Studies and surveys
replicate this conclusion.[4][5] Where money has been allo-

1. Albee, G. W., *Mental Health Manpower Trends*, New York: Basic
   Books, 1959.
2. Albee, G. W., Manpower Needs for Mental Health and the Role of
   Psychology. *The Canadian Psychologist*, 6a, 82–92, 1965.
3. Rieff, R., Mental Health Manpower and Institutional Change, in
   Brindman, A. J. and Spiegel, A. D. (editors), *Perspectives in Community Mental Health*, Chicago: Aldine Publishing Co., 1969, pp.
   635–649.
4. Glasscote, R. M. and Gudman, J. E., *The Staff of Mental Health
   Centers*, Washington: American Psychiatric Association and National Institutes of Mental Health, 1969.
5. National Institute of Mental Health, *The Nation's Psychiatrists*,
   Maryland: Public Health Service Publication No. 1885, 1969.

cated, up go the "help wanted" signs. Compacts are being established between neighboring centers to prevent person-nel raiding.[6] The buyers' market has generated a mental health personnel inflation of its own. The manpower squeeze seems inevitable and predictable. Some have antic-ipated this condition and have looked to new sources for manpower, while others have tried to create "model" pro-grams with special incentives to attract a disproportionate percentage of the manpower pool.

It would seem that the inexorable certainty of mathe-matics assures us that the goal of mental health services for everyone is as whimsical as is a chicken in every pot. How many people will go where before the money dries up may be the only rational question. Meanwhile, all those who have a stake in creating the ubiquitous "delivery of med-ical care" systems, declare that innovation and bold initia-tives will bridge the manpower chasm. To note the need for help and to be willing to experiment with new kinds of "caretaking personnel" is wise. To expect to be able to create a new manpower resource so that each 200,000 person catchment area will have a responsibly staffed mental health center is something else. When all is said and done, the difference between helping and meddling with the lives of others is not spanned by good intentions. Help-ing people with mental problems is very difficult work. Many different kinds of people, both trained and un-trained, can do this but many cannot. Because the trained have not been able to prove that their "therapie" accom-plishes more than would have occurred without them, any-one and everyone is having a hand at it. The untrained will

6. In the city of Philadelphia, eleven community mental health cen-ters are contiguous and cover the area of the entire city. The Forum, an organization loosely developed as a voluntary co-ordinating structure for the centers, with a membership of their directors, has developed guidelines and agreements as to person-nel transfers between centers. This over-the-counter attempt at control is often balanced by under-the-counter extras to attract needed personnel.

no doubt attempt to perpetuate themselves by also nimbly avoiding the test of outcome. No one dares entertain the thought, let along the possibility, that people simply are incapable of intentionally helping other people, or conversely that people cannot be intentionally helped. The testing of that hypothesis would run contrary to our innermost convictions about man's utility to man. And so we remain optimistically committed to the notion that men do help other men—but if only we knew how, and if only it proves to be statistically significant.

Whatever else it is, psychotherapy seems, to me at least, to possess the essential ingredients of Socratic dialogue.[7] Whether in groups, families, or in dyadic office encounters, someone who has lost or has never known himself truly, is being challenged, questioned, and engaged so as to rediscover or find that truth. The mutuality of the encounter is not equal. One participant seeks himself, while the other seeks to help. Two persons, equally in search of themselves, may come together, question and reason together, and may come closer to the truth. To call that psychotherapy is to make of that word, so great a tautology, that it be-

---

7. Scott Buchanan's conversations with Harris Wofford, Jr., published as Embers of the World (Santa Barbara: The Center for the Study of Democratic Institutions, 1970) touch on the use of Socratic dialogue in psychiatry. " . . . . . . the great insight of Socrates that every human being is of this kind. If you examine him, if he examines himself with the help of a dialectician, you and he will discover that he is like that, and if you go on, you will find that all men are like that: they have minds, can think, ask questions and answer them, discover who they are, what the world's about and a whole lot of things." And " . . . . . . Its aim, of course, is to bring about some actual integration but it tends to pull people to pieces and if it isn't carried through to real insight it can be very very demoralizing and destructive, extremely so. Following the argument wherever it leads may mean a very, very long route. It isn't a quick way to recover. It can be, but often it is a very distant thing. You know, even Socrates said—or Plato makes him say—that dialectic is a dangerous thing for young men." (p. 31—32).

comes utterly meaningless. A starting point then in this wilderness of therapeutic identity: there must be a difference between the role of patient (client or other "innovative" term) and the role of therapist (psychotherapist, intervener, or what have you).

There is, of course, a presumption in my having used the term psychotherapy at all in the foregoing discussion. In some quarters psychotherapy, as a concept, is quite passé to many who see behavior as more fundamentally a socially determined phenomenon. They walk with Durkheim, without apparently knowing him, and are liberated by an old view in modern trappings.[8] This confusion, about whether the delivery system is to deliver psychotherapy or is to deliver something else, lies at the heart of the manpower problem.

The critical point in all of this lies with the approach used to define a problem. With "sophisticated" thinking it is possible to "relate" any phenomenon to any other. The decision to visit a podiatrist can be related to the climate. The difference between relationship and causality is so frequently ambiguous that it is commonplace today to see and hear most problems described in the grand dimension.[9] Adolescent rebellion is related to the hydrogen

8. Robert A. Nisbet in *The Sociological Tradition*, (New York: Basic Books, Inc.: 1966) says of Durkheim: "It is instructive to note that in Durkheim the tables of individualism are turned. Where the individualist perspective had reduced all that was traditional and corporate in society to the hard and unchanged atoms of individual mind and sentiment, Durkheim, in diametrically opposite fashion, makes the latter manifestations of the former. We have thus a kind of reverse reductionism, one that takes some of the deepest states of individuality—for example, religious faith, the categories of the mind, volition, the suicidal impulse—and explains them in terms of what lies outside the individual." (p. 83).

9. The differences between relationship and causality would require a philosophic treatise to develop adequate understanding. They are part and parcel of the dilemma regarding the meaning of determinism that has confounded great thinkers for generations.

bomb; acne to the War in Vietnam; depression to poverty; suicide to materialism, and on and on. The desperate fear of being irrelevant in one's view of the world promotes a kind of reverse naiveté. A little bit of social determinism apparently is intoxicating to someone discovering it for the first time.

Although the foregoing may have seemed a diversionary diatribe, it is really at the heart of the manpower problem. What one defines as the problem for which one needs manpower obviously determines the quantity and quality of manpower required. "What are you going to do with all these people?" That is *the* priority question.

Guidelines for the resolution of this question are notably poor. The most obvious is the psychiatric nomenclature, newly revised in the Diagnostic and Statistical Manual II of the American Psychiatric Association. Here is a listing of "problems" generally considered to fall within the mental illness rubric and hence target material for a mental health center. The nomenclature has enormous influence in its orienting perspective and is medical in its approach. The problems are named from the historical preoccupation of psychiatry and neurology and so the list is predictably oriented towards individuals. To use this perspective is to be person-focused and the wedding of this perspective with a social determinism outlook leads to chaos. The call for a "psychosocial nomenclature" has long been unanswered.[10]

Nonetheless that is the available guideline, and scores of mental health caretakers have been trained with it as the syllabus. Innovative approaches which take on a strong social determinism flavor (either in causal explanations of behavior or in treatment approaches) become difficult to communicate. Methods of operation are rarely standardized because there is no standard grid (nomenclature) to provide a language. This is difficult enough when "profes-

10. Bahn, A. K., Need of a Classification Scheme for the Psychosocial Disorders. *Public Health Reports*, 80, 79–82, 1965.

sionals" are concerned but the situation becomes impossible when persons of little experience try to relate to these "innovative" programs. What happens is that problems are talked about in innovative terms but acted on as if the standard DSM-II nomenclature were the guide. A severely disturbed psychotic person may be discussed within a perspective which accounts for the influence of his family, his job, his economic status, his culture, the impinging social institutions etc., but the "treatment" is aimed at him with "drugs," "support," etc.

We come up against a sobering piece of reality. The "manpower problem" cannot even be discussed without first resolving the task identity problem. Traditional psychiatric tasks, *i.e.* focus on individuals, families or small groups, who demonstrate behavior as described and listed in DSM-II, are the most well developed. If a center is content to address itself to those tasks, then the manpower needs can be discussed. If a center wishes to broaden or redefine the tasks, then it must start with the recognition that types of manpower, training of manpower, job-task descriptions for manpower, and resources for manpower are issues that must remain unsettled for years and years to come.[11]

This chapter has two possible alternatives at this point. It can end, stating that until the tasks are sufficiently clear we can go no further, or it can continue, assuming that some centers may yet find the tasks in DSM-II sufficiently relevant to their goals, or that some centers will attempt to develop their own clarity as to tasks, manpower, and manpower training.

11. By "unsettled" I here refer to the type of closure one might hope for through broad concensus of professionals working throughout the field or by scientific discovery. Both consensus and discovery are far off. It is certainly feasible, however, (as will be argued throughout this book) for idosyncratic "working definitions" for all of these issues.

THE BASIC DISCIPLINES

Presumably, the mental health professions have developed their identity on the premise that they *know* something (be it ever so little) about human behavior. The sacred quartet of psychiatrist, psychologist, social worker and nurse (unalterably in that order) have earned their fundamental relevance to the mental health center, if not by accomplishment, at least by their intention. They have been the ones most ready to assume responsibility for treatment and come from a professional training more or less systematically ordered to prepare them for treatment tasks.

If one begins with these four professions and adopts an economy model of supply and demand, the shortages in such personnel is glaring. The professional therapist treating a patient-client (the so-called medical model) may have inherent theoretical problems but the major practical problem is that there are not enough therapists to go around. It is not uncommon to hear about the advantages of using non-professionals based on various ethnic and socio-cultural grounds. Usually, these are based on some variation of the noble savage theme, but most reasonable persons recognize that necessity has been the primary agent in the proliferation of non-professional, para-professional, and indigenous programs.[12] As Goldberg discovered in a study of the staff of a mental health center composed of professional and non-professional therapists,[13] both groups overwhelmingly would prefer a traditional profes-

12. There is considerable heat about the preferable use of indigenous workers over and above the use of professionals. I would prefer to avoid that debate until the rules of discourse are clearly drawn and the messianic naiveté of the inexperienced indigenous advocate is sufficiently exorcised.
13. Goldberg, D., personal communications from an as yet unpublished study done in 1970 at the Temple University Community Mental Health Center.

sional to treat members of their family if mental health care were needed.

There are two divergent paths which have been used in the utilization of the basic disciplines. One is based on their professional differences, while the other on their professional similarity. With the former, the patient and/or problem is divided into parts with a professional assigned to the part most nearly corresponding to his range of supposed expertise.[14] When the basic disciplines are oriented with their sameness in mind, it is assumed that any and all of them can provide "treatment" with considerable overlap in expertise. The former model, *i.e.* based on professional dissimilarity, is the more traditional team approach, whether it is being used in a hospital setting or outpatient setting. The latter mode, *i.e.* based on professional similarity, is the newer approach. It is based on a know-nothing humility by the psychiatrist and psychologist and bold initiation by the social worker and nurse.[15] This gives an illusory boost to the manpower pool since, instead of a four-man team focused on one problem, we have four persons focused on four problems.

The more traditional team approach has logic on its side. Patients and their problems seem naturally to fall into a differentiated analysis. There are behavioral components which spring from bodily organ systems, from psychological systems, from social contexts, and from cultural value systems. If a patient and his problem are approached from a comprehensive point of view, then the multiple variables in that approach could not be adequately handled by a solitary specialist—nor could we expect the ordinary solitary

14. This is similar to the distribution of labor principles as utilized by industry in the "assembly line" type of operation.

15. This is not to imply that the psychiatrists and psychologists are the truly omniscient and the social workers and nurses the truly uninformed. This model of work does break down the hierarchical relationship which has obtained in the past, however, and is able to do so because of the willingness of the various professionals to "play a new game."

"treater" to become a multidisciplinary specialist. Treatment by a solitary specialist demands problem parsimony not comprehensiveness.

When problem parsimony is the vogue, *i.e.* focusing on discrete, clearly limited behavioral phenomena, then the argument for a non-team approach is the strongest. The issue must be further clarified by the following axiom: Behavior analysis can be made comprehensive or it can be made parsimonious—at the discretion of the person performing the analysis. It follows then that one can pick limited goals in treatment—perhaps requiring less manpower—or one can pick broad goals in treatment—probably requiring more manpower. One is not *more noble* than the other. For every sophisticated, broad behavioral analysis, someone else can become more sophisticated and comprehensive.

There are certain explicit and implicit limits which devolve from the use of the sacred quartet. None of these professionals know how to build a building, stop a war or influence the interest rate . . . . at least not as function of their professional discipline. Their excursions into the domain of others will be short-lived, since megalomania does not long survive the gasses of reality.

But having sounded the conservative warning it remains to look further at the pitfalls of the team approach. The most important difficulty is a seldom appreciated basic discontinuity between the four disciplines. They do not fit together like a hand in a glove. Their identities and therefore their functions are not closely collaborative. The functions may fall in the same general area but the gaps between them are significant enough to make a true team approach difficult at best.

Let us try to illustrate the above. Consider a psychotic patient with hallucinations and delusions, who is able to live outside an institution. His behavior is not disruptive to others and he has a concerned family which tries to tolerate his behavior. He is poorly motivated for treatment and actively avoids any attempts to secure help from any quarter. His employer has exhausted his patience and has discharged the patient until such time as he shows himself to be free of mental disorder. The patient's children are beginning to show strained reactions at school to the surprise and consternation of their teachers.

Within the above description there are problems at many levels. As one looks at the situation he can organize his understanding of the problem in a variety of ways:

1. The problem of the individual with his psychotic symptoms.

2. The problem of the etiology of the psychotic episode.

3. The problem of a reluctant patient, unwilling to cooperate in a treatment sense.

4. The problem of the psychological stress to each family member by virtue of their attempts to maintain a psychotic member.

5. The problem of the educational difficulties being experienced by the children.

6. The problem of economic strain since the discharge of the patient from his place of employment.

7. The problem of the employer's lack of sensitivity in the assistance of a mentally ill employee.

In the interest of problem parsimony we could decide to focus on any one of the above problems. As the focus expands to two or more problems it becomes less likely that a single treater can make sufficient impact. If we consider all seven of the problem parts in need of "treatment," then who on the team shall do what? At first impulse we can state that the first part, *i.e.* the individual and his symptoms, should be approached by the psychiatrist. But why? If psychotherapy is intended, then presumably the psychiatrist or psychologist has the training and experience to intervene. And yet the "treatment" of psychotic in-patients is often performed by other professionals and even non-professionals. Well then, if chemotherapy is to be used, it is clearly the job of the psychiatrist. And yet, once a medical judgment has been made as to choice of drugs and dosage, is the psychiatrist the most appropriate person to see to its administration and its regular use?

This process of unraveling responsibility can be repeated for each problem part. The implications of this role discontinuity are documented in a recent field survey of eight community mental health centers which used a team approach.[16] In none of them was there a consistent relationship between a person's discipline and how he spent his time. This role diffusion has one predictable consequence: team work, if it is to be successful, must be based on task clarity (already discussed as poorly clarified) and manpower distributed in such a way so as to have each component of the total task dealt with by a competent person. Since neither of these conditions are systematically met, team work becomes a euphemistic term at best.

The point to all of this is simply to indicate that the sacred quartet does not necessarily a team make. At the risk of redundancy it must be stated that task clarity and role identity are *both* prerequisites to real team work.

INDIGENOUS VARIATIONS

One prominent innovation prompted by the emergence of community mental health centers, has been the use of non-professional persons in tasks heretofore reserved for the professional.[17] The so-called indigenous worker has been used in a great variety of ways, under varying circumstances, with variable motivation and after greater or lesser degrees of training. In some instances their role has been peripheral, with tasks of a rather menial sort.[18] In other instances their role has been much more dramatic and

16. Glasscote, R. M. and Gudman, J. E., op. cit. 1969.
17. Torrey, E. F.: The Case of the Indigenous Therapist, *Arch Gen Psychiat* 20: 365–373, 1969.
18. Several Philadelphia based community mental health centers use "indigenous" workers in marginal roles, above clerical status but below expeditors.

crucial to the treatment plan. Some centers use the indigenous worker as a primary therapist.[19] Other centers have developed expeditor roles for them or have used them as linkage people, *i.e.* providing a close monitor and enabling function as a patient moves from one caretaking agency to another.[20] The variations are many and experimentation in their use is still rather primitive.

Something consistent seems to emerge from the experiences of those who have worked closely with the indigenous workers. There is an abiding realization that many "mental health" tasks can be performed quite well by the indigenous worker. It is impossible to say what tasks they perform well because experience suggests that their ability is not a function of their "indigenousness," nor probably of their training, but rather a function of their own idiosyncratic interpersonal qualities.[21] This raises enormous problems for the efficient and effective use of the indigenous person. If in fact their role identity, to be effective, should be closely linked to their own personality strengths, then the selection process becomes crucial. The selection process and not the training experience is probably the priority issue. Most centers, although acknowledging the importance of selection, go into orbit over the need for training. The presumption is that given a grossly undifferentiated person to start with, shaping and training will make a differentiated mental health worker. It can be argued, however, that training is simply the icing on a pre-existing cake, and it is the cake that counts, *i.e.* the basic personality strengths.[22]

19. Lynch, M., Gardner, E. A., Felzer, S. B.: The Role of Indigenous Personnel as Clinical Therapists, *Arch Gen Psychiat* 19:428-434, 1968.
20. Hansel, N., Wodarczyk, M., Visotsky, H.: The Mental Health Expeditor, *Arch Gen Psychiat* 18:392, 1968.
21. A controlled study contrasting therapeutic outcome between professional therapists and indigenous therapists is yet to be done.
22. The same argument may be applied to the effectiveness of professional therapists as well, *i.e.* are they born more than they are trained?

The problem, of course, is not simply a matter of discovering the abilities already inherent in the indigenous worker but also fitting those abilities to appropriate tasks. Again, we do not have a helpful nomenclature of problem tasks and so the fitting of talent to task is very intuitive and grossly inefficient.

Does all this mean that the indigenous worker is not economically feasible as a manpower resource? The answer is yes . . . . with qualifications. At this point in time, the indigenous worker is not a sound economic venture, despite their uniformly poor pay. But it is not their fault. We have simply not developed the kind of organizational structures which use them to full advantage (nor have we for the sacred quartet). We have not developed a suitable nomenclature, based on problem phenomena and task parsimony, so as to be able to fit the talent to the task. Instead, we have assigned them to tasks often beneath their ability or over their head. We have multiplied the manpower drain by tight supervisory connections and redundant checks on their performance. Or we have left them to drift without adequate supervision or minimal checks.

Despite these problems, however, optimism should prevail. Important precedents have been set and consequent work will sharpen the focus and efficiency, and undoubtedly make an impact not only on psychiatry but on medicine in general.

A neglected aspect of the indigenous worker trend is its impact on the mental health establishment as a transmitter of culture and therefore as an instrument of organizational sensitivity. At this stage of the game, this contribution may be greater than that of a manpower resource. Community mental health centers have crossed many foreign borders. Not the least important of these is the border from affluence to poverty. It is ironic that professional training makes much use of "the poor" as objects of study but fails to get under the skin. We may be as prepared to take out a poor person's appendix as a rich one's, but we are not as prepared to talk to a poor person (and listen to him) as we are to understand an affluent person. In the "mental health" business, that is a deadly flaw.

The introduction of the indigenous worker into the organizational life of a mental health center carries with it the *chance* that the cultural ethos of that organization can be influenced. The chance may never be actualized if the indigenous person is placed in too peripheral a role. But given an important role, that person can bring the elements of the so-called culture of poverty into the organization's awareness. It can become organizationally sensitive. This bridge to reality is a critical part of any successful organization and keeps it from creating air conditioners for the Eskimos.

THE MULTIDISCIPLINARY SYSTEM: MAXIMUM FEASIBLE OVERLAP

If, at this point, the reader is somewhat confused, what with psychiatrists, psychologists, social workers, nurses and indigenous workers milling about, bumping into each other, then the point of this chapter will have been made. The time-study experts, who harass the industrial workers, but who somehow push the company into productive efficiency, would have a field day with the economic absurdity of our pseudo-team approach. The multidisciplinary system is really an undisciplined non-system more often than not. If the reader feels that it is unfair to level so harsh a criticism without an accompanying alternative plan, he is only partially justified. The alternative has already been stated. It is not a new structural arrangement but rather a call for conceptual clarity at the level of task identification. Saying that we or they shall do "psychotherapy" or "give support" or "environmental manipulation" is not enough. What are the parts of these operations? What are the task definitions? Until or unless we make headway in this direction, the use of the multidisciplinary model will continue to be a haphazard and expensive illusion.

ADAPTATION AND A PSYCHOSOCIAL NOMENCLATURE

As has been noted, our current nomenclature fails us in certain key areas. There are generally useful implications for treatment which derive from the various nosologic categories. Some of these categories are based on formal test results with attached presumptive etiology (Mental Retardation) and some on etiologic organic changes (Senile Dementia, Alcoholic Psychosis, Psychosis associated with intracranial infection, etc.). Some nosologic categories are based on phenomenologic syndromes without any etiologic assumptions (Schizophrenia, Affective Disorders). Some categories are based on principles of mental dynamics with neither phenomenologic standards nor etiologic assumptions (Hysterical Neurosis, Phobic Neurosis). Some categories are based on selected personality characteristics with neither dynamic, nor etiologic assumptions (Personality Disorders, Sexual Deviation). Some categories are based on discrete organ function with neither etiologic, nor characterologic nor dynamic assumptions (Psychophysiologic Disorders). Some categories are based on developmental theory with specific life cycle relevance but without clear phenomenologic standards, nor etiologic assumptions, nor characterologic assumptions (Transient Situational Disturbances).

In summary DSM-II is a potpourri of categorization without a consistent frame of reference. It mixes phenomenology, etiology, characterology, dynamic theory, functionalism, and developmental theory in a dyspepsic soup. It demands a high degree of sophistication from those who would use it as a guide for behavioral organization. It gives little help to those who would use it as a guide for treatment or intervention. This shortcoming is therefore most obvious with less sophisticated mental health workers who have an interventional role to play.

6

Anyone who has had experience in working with sophisticated mental health professionals will also appreciate that these sophisticated professionals use the nomenclature in very arbitrary and idiosyncratic ways. Their use of the nomenclature tends to be administrative and has little to do with how they conceptually organize their patient's problem and treatment.

The interventionally relevant nosology must follow certain laws of logic. If it is to follow one or more frames of reference, then these must be made explicit at the outset and must be carried throughout the nosologic system. The most advantageous frame of reference, for interventional purposes, is the etiologic. If we can know the cause of selected behavior, then our intervention is focused immediately. We may not have resources or the technology within our treatment to influence the cause, but we can at least come as close as possible to influencing the cause. And so an interventional nosology must place ultimate priority on etiology, when it is known.

It is my contention that one can construct a useful nosology incorporating principles of etiology, phenomenology, characterology and functionalism. A full explanation and development of these concepts are beyond the scope of this work but let me at least provide a broad outline so as to at least orient the reader to my general meaning.

We must start by placing the above four perspectives (etiology, phenomenology, characterology, and functionalism) within a comprehensive frame of reference. We need a concept general enough to subsume these four perspectives and yet sufficiently empiric so as to be more than a philosophic abstraction. This concept, around which the four perspectives are organized, is that of adaptation. The durable force which supports adaptation as our central concept is its position as the fundamental ecologic process of living organisms. To "adapt" is to bring two contiguous systems into dynamic relationship, with the "survival" of both systems as ultimately determining the extent and nature of the relationship.

This principle, whether seen in the context of evolutionary process or in the narrower dimension of psychosocial relationship is, at all times, operative in determining the behavior of both contiguous systems. One of the basic realities at the very heart of evolution is its appreciation of the mutuality of organism and context. On the one hand, there is ample evidence that organisms begin with a given structural constitution from which eventually flow various functions. But on the other hand, there is also ample evidence that, over a substantial temporal span, the challenges of the organism's context provide impetus, through natural selection, for structural changes and consequent new functions. This is, essentially, the process of adaptation, i.e. a process where structure determines function, but where, simultaneously, the context's demand for a new function changes structure to permit new function. In this sense, evolutionary adaptation is at once a resonating equilibrium between structure and context. This can be compared to the acorn-oak, or chicken-egg pseudo-dilemmas. Weiss, from his biologic focus, refers to this as the "duality of fitness."[23] He differentiates between "evolutionary mechanisms" which derive from a "pre-design" and "on-the-spot adjustments" which are responsive to the demands of the external.

Although adaptation, when considered in this historical and evolutionary sense, is of a different order than when considered on the individual human level, there are certain common features. As ontogeny recapitulates phylogeny, the individual human features of adaptation recapitulate the evolutionary features of adaptation. This thread of conceptual consistency from the phylogenetic to the ontogenetic further supports the use of adaptation as our central concept and allows for its use at any of the general

23. Weiss, Paul: "The Biological Basis of Adaptation," in Romano, John (ed.), *Adaptation*, Ithaca: Cornell University Press, 1949.

system levels of organization. In a real sense it is the adaptive process between molecule and atom, between cell and organ, between psyche and context that is the unifying process from which all behavior is derived.

Piaget, from an epistemologic and developmental viewpoint, also sees adaptation in a dual sense.[24] He refers to "accommodation," *i.e.* the work of the organism's structures upon the external, and to "assimilation," *i.e.* the influence of the external upon the structures of the organism.

This dual aspect of adaptation, *i.e.* a dynamic mutuality of organism and context, is very germane when one is attempting to develop a systematic frame of reference at the level of relationship between the psychologic and the social.

These implications, which follow upon the use of adaptation as a central referent, make it conceptually possible to consider behavior in a way that is not possible if we were to think of such terms as "normal," "equilibrium," "conscious," "function," etc. The conceptual limitations are based on the fact that with these latter terms we already possess an understanding which, both connotatively and denotatively, preclude our consideration of an *organism-context fit through time*. This is a critical point. Although it can be argued that equilibrium-disequilibrium denotes an organism-context relationship, it does so without conveying a sense of time. It does not permit one to appreciate the reality of the change (or evolution) of the organism's structures (through time) as accomplished by the influence of the context (nor the reciprocal of this). When human behavior is seen as a variant of adaptedness, its richness of variation becomes logically acceptable.

It follows that since adaptation is a dualistic concept its referential points may come from two sources, *i.e.* the

24. Flavell, John H.: *The Developmental Psychology of Jean Piaget*, Princeton: D. Van Nostrand Co. Inc., 1963.

organism and/or its context. Inherent in the organism is a biologic system of signalling unadaptedness. Whether this is seen as May's existential angst,[25] or Freud's primary and secondary anxiety,[26] is largely a matter of varying primary focus and different assumptive belief systems. We may safely state that unadapted states often stimulate an affective response within the organism. At the core, *anxiety* is the referent but this affect may immediately change to derivative states of depression, guilt, shame, anomie, etc. and into Erikson's signs of life-cycle troubles.[27] But as has been noted often, affective concomitants are not readily apparent in certain "obvious" maladapted states, as in the so-called personality disorders or in the chronic schizophrenias. The essential difference here is that the reference points come not from the organism's affective signal but from the criteria of the external world. It is society reacting to organismic behavior which is at odds with its own socio-cultural norms. The signal is, in a sense, a group affect as the group attempts to reject the intrusion of the individual. The individual is an unaccommodated "foreign-body" to the group, as the group (*i.e.* context) may be an unassimilated "foreign-body" to the individual. Society says that these behaviors are not suitable because they conflict with its own criteria of adequate role performance. This is, in a real sense, an arbitrary distinction, since sociology and anthropology tell us convincingly that what is considered mal-adaptive by one socio-cultural group may not be considered mal-adaptive in another. Masserman's comments about sexuality and its cultural variations with attendant variability in "normal" or acceptable behavior is a striking example.[28] The influence of the Victorian west-

25. May, Rollo: *Existence*, New York: Basic Books, Inc., 1958.
26. Freud, S.: *The Problem of Anxiety*, New York: Norton, 1936.
27. Erikson, E. H.: *Identity and the Life Cycle*, Psychological Issues, 1:18–164, 1959.
28. Masserman, Jules H.: in Frontiers of Clinical Psychiatry, 3:18, September 15, 1966.

ern culture of the 19th Century upon Freud's thought is clear in the primacy he accorded sexuality (or, more correctly, its repression). If similar principles of theory were applied in today's sexually pre-occupied world, we might end up with a completely obverted core concept, *i.e.* of basic asexuality with defense through sexual preoccupation.

Moving now from this broad base, which I feel is inherently necessary, we arrive at a position which is essentially as follows: Behavior is a reflection of multiple dynamic states between contiguous systems, be they at molecular levels of organization or at psycho-context levels of organization, all of which are occurring simultaneously. These dynamic states tend towards a resolution of conflict which is inherent in the unending confrontation between, for example, the organism's structures with their attending functions and the environment's structures with their attending demands upon the organism. The resolution or *adaptation* is thus *mutually* determined by all interacting systems and so mal-adaptations are likewise mutually defined.

We now must integrate our four perspectives (etiology, phenomenology, characterology, and functionalism) within the fabric of this concept of adaptation. That which we wish to categorize must be clear. Our nosology must be focused not on adaptation but on mal-adaptation. We are interested in formulating a nomenclature based on failures in adaptation. Again we must make a distinction. There are failures in adaptation that should be left untouched by aggressive therapists. To a great degree we grow in maturity and competence by being allowed to struggle with the challenges of the adaptive process. To be relieved of this difficult and often painful work may be to preclude future autonomy. And so it is reasonable to differentiate mal-adaptation from the point of view of interventional need. I prefer to think in terms of adaptive dissonance and adaptive disorganization.

We may define adaptive dissonance as the continuous gradient between the organism and its context which works against adaptation. Having succeeded in adapting to the demands of a new job simply means fulfilling some of those demands by developing some personal routines and strategies but the job will always present new tasks and demands requiring new responses. This adaptive dissonance keeps us working at the perpetual task of adaptation.

We may define adaptive disorganization as a state of adaptive dissonance so marked in the degree of gradient that adaptive attempts become counter-productive and the gradient is either fixed or enlarged.

This is how our nosologic schema looks at this point:

I. Behavior (as a function of human adaptation)
   A. Successful Adaptation
   B. Mal-adaptation
      1. Adaptive Dissonance
      2. Adaptive Disorganization

The nomenclature begins at "Adaptive Disorganization." Our next task is to focus on each of the two key variables in the adaptive process, the organism and the nature of its relationship to its context. We focus on the organism by designating its durable personality, (characterology). We focus on the organism's contextual relationship by specifying the behavioral phenomenology and by specifying the degree of functional discongruence between the organism and its context (functionalism). The functional concept has often been used with social competence or social adequacy scales. If we have information as to the cause (etiology) of the adaptive disorganization then we can so specify. Often the cause can simply be a basic disparity between the adaptive repertoire of the organism (characterology) and the adaptive challenge of the context.

We can now visualize the nosologic schema as follows:

I. Adaptive Disorganization
   A. Phenomenology (including signs and symptoms)

B. Characterology
C. Functionalism
D. Etiology

The schema needs quantification. That is a fundamental requirement since it can then give a cleavage indicator between adaptive dissonance and adaptive disorganization and it can also serve to mark increments of improvement or worsening. The implications of a quantifiable nosology are vast and again beyond the scope of this work.

Let us try to apply the foregoing to a clinical problem:

Mrs. Smith, a forty-year-old married woman complains of feeling tense and irritable and is periodically overcome with tearfulness and depression. She has become increasingly critical of her husband of twenty two years and he has reacted with anger and frustration at her persistent change. She has gradually fallen behind in the upkeep of her home and she has been unable to socialize with her long-standing friends. Further exploration reveals that she developed these symptoms shortly after her daughter's marriage and subsequent move from the home.

Mrs. Smith had always been a busy, outgoing person with many friends. She took great pleasure in these relationships and was considered a natural leader and effective organizer. Her pace was often frenetic. One characteristic of note was her great sensitivity to criticism, even when this was of a minor sort. She could readily withdraw in such a situation and might become apathetic and self-critical. She seemed to have a basic low self-esteem which she compensated for through activities designed to bring her reassuring positive feed-back from her environment. But her greatest sense of worth had been gradually developed in the relationship with her daughter. They had always been close and could confide totally with one another. The daughter's marriage had been anticipated and Mrs. Smith was the driving force in planning and implementing the marital celebrations. She fully approved of her new son-in-law.

This case could be diagnosed by the DSM-II in a variety of ways. Some would focus on the symptomatic expression of affect. The most likely diagnostic choice would be "Depressive Reaction." Some would add subsidiary phrases like "with anxiety." Another diagnostician might choose to focus on the situational implications of the problem and so make the diagnosis "Adjustment Reaction of Adult Life." It is even conceivable that one might choose to focus on her basic personality type and attribute her problem to a characterologic decompensation.

Regardless of the ultimate choice, the diagnosis itself gives little helpful information. The planning of treatment depends on a further recitation of historical facts, presumed dynamics, personality characteristics and "strengths" and so on. In the hands of a lesser trained mental health worker the rubric "Depressive Reaction" or "Adjustment Reaction of Adult Life" is nearly worthless.

Using our adaptation schema we might develop something like the following:

I. Adaptive Disorganization—Acute
    A. Depression (grπ)—and anxiety (grπ)
    B. Low self-esteem syndrome (compensated)
    C. Functionally decompensated
        marital-household (grπ)
        social (grπ)
    D. Compensatory esteem deficiency.

Essentially what we have done is to replace a single phrase rubric with a systematic outline giving the salient features of a behavioral analysis from phenomenologic, characterologic, functional and etiologic perspectives. The quantitative designations are without foundation in the example and depend upon a well-articulated system of criteria weighting.

This section cannot stand alone without a great deal more elaboration. But it was not my intention to provide more than an orienting statement so that my oft-repeated criticism of our present nomenclature could have the company of at least one alternative approach.

PROFESSIONALISM

With the new self-effacement that seems inherent in many community psychiatrists a cult of anti-professionalism and anti-intellectualism has been bred in many of the more "innovative" mental health centers. It is not surprising to find agnosticism following on the heels of frustration. In a field as ill defined as community mental health, it follows almost absolutely that failures and hence frustration abound. Even the most discretely defined human problem is difficult to influence systematically. Given a tendency to vacillate between problem parsimony and problem expansion (as is the way in most "innovative" programs) the prospects of successful systematic intervention drop precipitously. As a consequence, systematic approaches become undermined. The systematic approach frustrates and so a flying-by-the-seat-of-our-pants approach is generated. Since neither A, B, nor C seem to work, let's throw out D through Z as well.

This attitude fits in well with the prevailing anti-intellectual air in America. There is a current penchant for immersion into a feeling world, through sensitivity groups, drugs, encounters and confrontations and a rejection of plodding rationalism. An aura of nobility has attached to emotionalism and one of crass self-seeking has attached to rationality. The "innovative" mental health center has an enormous need to "be with it" and to avoid "traditionalism," "rigidity," the "medical-model," the mayor and the devil. With subtle and yet devasting effect, these negative attitudes have also attached to "professionalism." Curiously enough, some of the most influential leaders of this anti-professionalism are professionals themselves.

What seems to have happened is that many professionals, originally intent on providing help of sorts to distressed and disadvantaged persons, have given up this goal and in its stead are looking for love from these same distressed, disadvantaged persons. It has been a rapid run from noblesse oblige to mea culpa. The professional has warranted his share of criticism in perpetuating oppressive institutions but not because of his professionalism. When guilty, it has been because of his human frailty and the self-seeking qualities he shares with all men, professional and non-professional alike. Being a professional means being knowledgeable and proficient in selected tasks. It will be the end of the mental health center and any other institution when they no longer have persons who have knowledge and competence for the needed tasks. The quality of the man who is accredited is a more crucial variable than the accreditation itself.

Professionalism, with or without accreditation, should be the top priority in manpower design. The use of people who know what they are doing and why is old-fashioned, traditional and so very important.

chapter 4

ADMINISTRATIVE STRUCTURES AND PROCESSES:

Democratic Imperialism

The ultimate frustration for many doctors and for psychiatrists in particular is the responsibility of "administration." To be an administrator is to push papers, sign your name endlessly, harass employees, balance a budget, agonize over a blueprint, recruit reluctant staff candidates, fire incompetents, apologize to one's superiors, and perform countless other non-medical operations. When a doctor does in fact find himself doing the above in his "administrator's" hat he has fallen prey to an old organizational species, "octopus ineffectus." The self-fulfilling prophecy haunts its prophet. The bound-up administrator tied the knots himself.

Levinson and Klerman made a useful distinction that goes to the core of the administrative muddle.[1] They dif-

1. Levinson, D. J. and Klerman, G. L.: The Clinician–Executive, *Psychiatry* 30:3, 1967.

ferentiated the executive from the implementer and characterized each role from within a medical perspective. Some men are meant to plan, conceptualize, order priorities, and assume ultimate organizational responsibilities. Others are meant to implement these plans, and to maintain organizational viability. The former are the executives and the latter are the implementers. The experience, training and talents of each are different although occasionally some men are good at both. It is pathognomonic of a disordered organization to have a blurring of the executive and implementer roles. The executive who personally examines the time clock records as a matter of routine, or who has all of his personnel relate directly to him, is neither an executive nor an implementer. He is a muddler. Unfortunately medical administrators tend to fall into this blurred role by virtue of their lack of administrative training and because of their characteristic over-reliance on authority. The autocratic role, so efficient in the surgical suite, can be quite unproductive in the manager's office.

PARTICIPATORY AND NON-PARTICIPATORY OPTIONS

There is much in the dichotomy of leading and being led that feeds naturally into a great variety of dissimilar events, from a baseball game to a revolution. A revolution attempts to overthrow a leader. But a revolution, if not led, will be fruitless. So the nobility of a revolution does not lie in its opposition to any leadership but rather in its opposition to certain leadership. Presumably then it is sufficiently noble to be led under certain conditions. It doesn't take a political scientist to point out that leadership has its limits and those limits are set by those who are led. The degree to which they experience a sense of participation in the determination of their behavior is often the critical element in their toleration of their leaders.

And so it is in organizations, including and perhaps especially in mental health centers. There is a vital balance to be struck between the leader and the led so that their relationship to each other, and hence ultimately their joint relationship to their goals and methods, will be mutually creative and effective. But this balance is seldom achieved as a stable phenomenon. It is more likely a transient or episodic event interposed between periods of oligarchy and anarchy. Which is dominant for how long and how often gives an organization its personality, its strength or its weakness.

In a mental health center, goals and methods are at a level of abstraction that resists the mechanization of an automobile factory. Although much that has been written here has been a plea for specification and explicitness, the state of our cumulative knowledge leaves us necessarily in a position where the gaps are filled in with dedication, commitment, good will, common sense, intuition and some altruism. We do not build automobiles in a mental health center and so our product is not as immune to the above sentiments as is the cold polished steel of a new Ford. You can give orders until you are blue in the face, and they may all be followed, but that still may leave an enormous gap between goals and outcome.

The point to all of this is that the organization's success is dependent in great measure on what may vaguely be called morale and that in turn is influenced greatly by the successful mix of leadership and followership; which again brings us to the concept of participation.

Inherent in the meaning of participation is the aspect of shared experience, and shared followership. It is, like so many other words, a slippery one to pin down. There is a continuity of meaning within it which extends from minimal to maximal participation. Which dose is appropriate for which person is a tempting question but one which cannot be answered easily. Participation is too often thought of as a piece of the power without any necessary piece of the responsibility. It is within this neat equation of power and responsibility that the working out of how much participation should occur. If a situation is such that there is no way to share the responsibility, then there should be no way to share the power. If I am to operate on you—and the result of that operation will be charged or credited to me—then I would be a fool to turn the knife over to the aide and urge him to do the cutting. Now if you informed me that I could use my judgment in deciding who should cut but that the responsibility was still mine, I might risk giving the knife to another surgeon whose competence I trusted. The lesson from all of this is to see that there is a beginning point in the assignment of responsibility. A federal granting agency does not give its largesse to 200 people and say "you are all responsible for the performance of your organization." It says instead, "you, Mr. or Dr. X are responsible for the performance of that organization, and we will talk to you, (not to your 200 people) when we have questions about performance." When things go wrong and all hell breaks loose, where does the passing of the buck stop? If it stops with you, then you are where we must start in talking about participation and responsibility.

The responsible person should be an eager participant. If he is not, then he should not be in that job. If you tell Dr. X that he is to be responsible for the out-patient department, he should become an active participant in decision making about that out-patient department. If he is unwilling to participate in those decisions or is prevented from participating by rigidity from above, then the out-patient department is headed for big trouble. If we assume that Dr. X is responsible and actively involved in decision making about his department then he is a potential asset to the organization. Whether he is *actually* an asset depends on the judgment he exercises and upon his ability to make those persons working in his department responsible for their performances and collaterally, participants in decisions about their department and their work.

This could be incorrectly read as a call for anarchy or, in more current jargon, "everyone doing his own thing." It is not intended that way. Responsibility is intrinsically a relative concept. Everyone is not, nor could they be, responsible for everything. An organization, like a mental health center, has to be first thought of in terms of its goals. If it has none that are clearly stated and unambiguous, then we need proceed no further. Responsibility and participation in the service of nothing is nothing. But assuming an organization starts with purpose or goals, then these provide the ultimate guideline for all those who would share in the responsibility and in the pursuit of those goals. The highest level of responsibility is set (or at least, should be) before the organization is more than an idea. From that point on the diffusion of responsibility is passed downward by the decision of those at the highest level. To protect themselves they must be careful about how the process unravels. It is axiomatic to the concept of a trust (the trustee) that primary allegiance be paid to discrete goals. If it is in the interest of those goals to distribute various limited quantities of responsibility, then it should be done. But it is always done at the risk of the trustee, *i.e.* at the risk of the person or persons *ultimately entrusted* with the task of achieving the stated goals.

This gets worked out even further as we pass upwards in the maze of responsibility-participation equations. The trustee is responsible ultimately to the highest levels of public trust. We then get lost in the ascending connections to laws, governments and elected officials. This may seem a rather constipated way to get to a basic premise, but the clearest way between two points is not always a straight line.

The premise, as related to an organization like a community mental health center, is as follows: maximum efficiency in the service of organizational goals is directly proportional to the clarity of responsibility and degree of participation at the level of every employed person.

The remaining ambiguity in all of this may be in trying to understand what is meant by maximal participation.

The only possible way to clarify this is to state that processes like responsibility and participation must have a starting point and ending point. Spell out the responsibility and spell out the limits of participation. That spelling out must come from above. It is wisdom to listen to advice from below. It is judgment that decides which advice to follow and which to reject. It is irresponsibility which sets policy from the bottom up.

RULES OF CLOSURE: DECISION MAKING

Except for the rhetorical type, when a question arises, it may be presumed that an answer is desired. Questions and answers go together. Even if we don't know *the* answer to a question, a reasonable answer is "we don't know." An unanswered question generates anger, confusion and acting out. Have you every asked someone a question and had him ignore it? It is hard enough to swallow your pride and reveal your ignorance by asking the question in the first place, but then to have it left dangling in the air is like having your toupee pulled off. It is in the nature of an organization to generate questions. It is not in the nature of an organization to generate answers. There is a tendency to avoid answers or at least to complicate them, multiply them and to make them so ambiguous as to avoid closure.

It is the need for closure that starts a question. Closure moves towards a unity of understanding if not agreement. When there are many people working towards common goals, then it is imperative that closure be a characteristic of the organization. How the questions get answered, *i.e.* who has the information (in questions of fact) or who has the authority (in questions of responsibility) is not the point. Here the issue is not how but rather why and when questions must be answered.

We have already alluded to one reason why questions should be answered. To avoid answering is to generate anger. This may not be explosive, open anger but it is anger nonetheless. Again, to answer "I don't know" is an honest and therefore acceptable answer. It is much less likely to generate anger than the talking around, over and under the issue. The latter is born of deception and the hearer rarely fails to attribute the non-answer to cowardice or deception.

Another reason for closure is that there can be enormous communication foul-ups if questions are left to 200 people to answer. That may mean 200 different answers and when there are that many loose answers lying around, people will hear those they wanted to hear. It is a standard ploy of the organizational apologist, faced with an inefficient operation, to blame faulty communications for the problem. His explanation is that "communication *systems* are so complicated by nature that we haven't quite developed a good one in our organization." While it may be true that the maintenance of proper communication is difficult, it is often more true that various responsible persons in the organization have *avoided* answering legitimate questions raised by other persons from either above or below. If there is an insistence on closure at the top, then this will permeate the organization downwards and allow persons at all levels of responsibility to promote closure. If higher level persons do not allow closure at the lowest possible level, then these unanswered questions will constantly be drifting upward requiring an inordinate amount of time and energy from inappropriate people. The greater the tendency for questions to remain unanswered and the greater the trend towards upward drift, the greater the communication problem and the greater the organizational inefficiency.

It may very well be *better* to have questions answered incorrectly than not answered at all. An incorrect answer may be corrected later without paying the price of communication disorder. When a question arises there are several alternatives. If it is a question of fact, then either the answer is known or not known. If the facts are available but not immediately, so then the first answer is to state that we *will get* the final answer. The point is that a question is responded to with the clear communication that if the answer is not immediately available, then there will be a direct process leading either to the answer or the unequivocal statement that the information is not available, meaning no answer is possible. If an answer is possible—even if several intervening processes must come first —then the question should be answered immediately by spelling out how we shall get to the final answer.

THE COMMITTEE: BACKBONE OF THE INVERTEBRATE

Someone once said that a camel is a horse designed by a committee. Considering the fact that camels do pretty well in the inhospitable clime of the desert, that statement may be a compliment rather than an insult. What seems so disagreeable about a committee is that it compromises one's sense of autonomy. Somehow a consensus is the product of a committee and not the cool, crisp, devastating plan of a solitary genius. Since we all know that we are that genius, under the restraint of "the organization," it is aggravating to submit to this collective nit picking.

Despite our impulses to the contrary, many questions are best answered after they have been subjected to the assault of a committee. No committee should be formed unless there is a question to be asked of it and no committee should be asked a question if we are not prepared to hear its answer.

In a community mental health center there is a predictable mix of people. Doctors, psychologists, social workers, nurses (note the order) and others come together with more differences than similarities. These are differences which are ingrained to a large extent because of prior education and training and the biases that led them to choose their various disciplines in the first place. Working together will not be easy. The working together in committee can be one of the real role—model experiences which leads to an understanding of how each thinks and operates. It is not the same as working together in the real tasks of mental health care but that is to its advantage. In the work-a-day world where each discipline pursues its objectives along certain well-developed guidelines, there is a tendency to hide beneath professional prerogatives. "That's my job, not yours!" "No, that's his job, not mine!" But in the committee, if properly chaired, and if properly charged with a discrete task, people can relate to problems and learn the task of collective problem solving.

Beyond the experiential value in committee work it is clear that many issues arise which require a concerted in-depth approach. These are issues that cannot be resolved in the ordinary day-to-day line responsibilities of staff. It is important to spread the committee work assignments throughout the staff, from top to bottom both for the experiential value to the committee members, and to provide as much opportunity as possible for wise people to contribute. There are more gems of wisdom buried down the personnel line than most leaders realize.

INTERDISCIPLINARY COOPERATION

There are two aphorisms which apply when considering interdisciplinary cooperation: "Don't build an organization on heroism," and "Don't build an organization on love." Neither heroism nor love will make cooperation between disciplines. Heroes wear out and love is fickle. Professionals have been trained to have a perspective and each discipline reinforces its own peculiar perspective to the virtual exclusion of others.

In the behavioral sciences, interdisciplinary approaches have had a long history of currency.[2,3] But they have not

2. Sherif, M. and Sherif, C. W.: *Interdisciplinary Relationships in the Social Sciences*, Chicago: Aldine Publishing Company, 1969.
3. There have been attempts to institutionalize interdisciplinary research in problems of mental health. The Mental Health Research Institute at the University of Michigan represents such an attempt.

had a long history of success. Institutes for interdisciplinary research as well as interdisciplinary practice have succumbed to disciplinary megalomania.[4] They will work together and on the surface may seem to enjoy it. But when you strip away the personal relationships that bind these co-workers and leave their professionalism, you are left with a detente—as cool as the cold war.

If you desire an interdisciplinary organization, then it *must be worth their while* to work together. That means that the organization must place a high priority on the need for the idiosyncratic task for each discipline. The work of a social worker cannot be window dressing for the *more important* work of the psychiatrist. The goal structure of the organization must state goals which relate specifically to the input of the separate disciplines. And realistically, why bother to include various disciplines in your organization if you do not have tasks for which they alone are presumably prepared. If you don't really believe that is so, then do not bother to hire them in the first place.

Some community mental health centers have done away with disciplinary chiefs and have urged that professionals discard their disciplinary allegiance and work for the team.[5] That is a typical conclusion of the highest level executive, secure in his tenure, salary and prerogatives. But to a line person, faced with the problems of patients to start with, and then the unmentioned pecking order between disciplines, the unmentioned prestige differences, the unmentioned salary disparities and the unmentioned expectation differences—the call to renounce one's discipline is a call for heroism and love. It means throwing out

4. Campbell, D. T.: Ethnocentrism of Disciplines and the Fish-scale Model of Omniscience, in Sherif, M. and Sherif, C.: *Interdisciplinary Relationships in the Social Sciences,* Chicago: Aldine Pub. Co., pp. 328–348, 1969.

5. Several large community health centers in Philadelphia have insisted on primary responsibility to team leaders (of varying disciplinary background) and some have gone further by refusing to allow the development of any intra-disciplinary hierarchy.

the union card, credentials and diploma. Many new workers have been willing to go along with this in the service of innovation and excitement—but as with many a novelty grown tired, it will wear out.

The job is to blend various disciplines, not blur them. Social psychology did not arise from the grafting of a sociologist to a psychologist. It emerged as a new discipline with its own perspective, theory, method and identity. It rendered obsolete neither sociology nor psychology.[6]

INCENTIVE AND THE CORPORATE MODEL

People are willing to march to a variety of drums. But some drums are more appealing than others. In medical service, in its many varied forms, the drums to which people march are not the loud or exciting ones. To be willing to work in the medical organization (and here I will exclude the physician) a person must be willing to earn less, tolerate more, and advance slowly if at all.[7] That set of conditions is not designed to attract the most competent of people. If by circumstance and luck competent people are in the medical organization, chances are they will not stay there long. The incentives are poor, so why should they? If a medical institution has a sterling reputation for excellence, the credit quickly goes to the top (usually to an articulate physician). If the lesser staff can get their kicks from reflected glory, they may stay but don't count on it. So if they can't be payed competitively and they do not sense appreciation when their work leads to excellence, there will be a high personnel turnover and a steady decrease in the average level of competence.

How do you reverse this process? By being clear in your thinking, honest in your declarations and bold in your perspective. If people work best when they are pursuing

6. Allport, G.: Six Decades of Social Psychology, in *The Person In Psychology*, Boston: Beacon Press, pp. 28–42, 1968.
7. I exclude the physician because he has invariably fared rather well in an economic sense, especially when contrasted with his non-medical confreres within the same health organization.

noble goals, and when they can sniff success in that pursuit, and when they are being rewarded for their competence (not simply for filling a job slot) with *(a)* money and *(b)* recognition, then get people to work best by setting up those conditions.

We have had occasion to talk about goals a number of times already. The point to be made (again) is that goals must be stated in such a language and with such clarity that it will be possible for most normal men to decide whether they have been achieved or not. If a symposium of abstract theorists is required to debate the nature of your goals and the degree to which your organization achieved them, then you can be assured that the people in your mental health center will not know what the center *is really* supposed to be doing and whether it is succeeding at that nebulous task. Don't say that your goal is the provision of quality psychiatric service, or the provision of mental health, or an attack on mental illness. Those are words for the poet.

Once the organization knows what it's supposed to be doing it has something against which it can test its performance. And the component units as well as the individual persons can be evaluated in terms of their contribution to the attainment of those goals. Personnel evaluations based on such items as "level of information available" are fine for schools but not for mental health centers. "How many patients improved while under this person's care?" is a more meaningful question, providing "improved" is defined in unambiguous and measurable terms.

The problem of reward for competence is the least understood. Sometimes it means a pat on the back. Sometimes it may mean a complimentary statement in a group meeting. But more than these haphazard devices, recognition should be part of a visible system. Have you ever seen the large prominent chart hanging in an auto salesroom, listing the salesmen in rank order? Well that's not what I have in mind, but it's headed in the right direction.

Goals must be translated into numbers, even if you have to create a symbolic translator to tell you what the numbers mean. The organization must have an accurate intra-organizational reporting system which tells the story "how we are doing." People have to be able to see where they are in that report, where their unit is in that report and where their boss is in that report. The payoff in terms of recognition follows logically. The biggest problem of course is getting a *comprehensive* and *accurate* reporting system into operation.[8] The process of working towards such a system can be one of the most rewarding experiences that staff can have since it will force pious fluff to the test and may lead some people to find out what the business is all about.

The reinforcement of excellence by the use of money may not be Pavlovian but it has a long tradition of effectiveness. Why it isn't characteristic of medical organizations is probably due most of all to the solo entrepreneurial characteristic of the physician. He is not an organization man and he usually knows very little about what makes them tick. He has had sufficient recognition and financial reward and so has not been motivated to make economic sense out of a medical organization. The victims of this situation have been the "lesser" personnel of the medical organizations but more importantly the entrapped consumers who are dependent on the medical organization's product. Have you been in a hospital lately?

The other basic problem of course is that medical organizations rarely make money. They are constantly in the red.

Most organizations start out with the premise that they must take in more money (or its equivalent) than they pay out. That is the profit motive. The profit is then used to beef up the organization so that it will be in a better

8. Beck, I. C.: Record-keeping and Research, in Grunebaum, H. (edit.): *The Practice of Community Mental Health*, Boston: Little, Brown and Company, 1970.

position to make more profit, and so on it goes. A wise organization uses some of those profits as incentive bonuses for persons in the organization. That is the reward system to keep the organization sharp. The key to the whole system is the consumer (or customer). He must like the product and be willing to pay the price for it. In an affluent culture, the money is there. The market is determined by the need for the product. Consumer satisfaction keeps the whole thing working.

But in the medical world of the mental health center, if the governmental subsidy is reduced, the floor caves in and everyone says "I told you so." Something is wrong with an organization whose product is so poorly thought of that no one is willing to pay the price of production. If the governmental agency is your life-line to existence, then do not be surprised when the bubble bursts. If your product is too expensive for the consumer, then you must work to lower the price. If you have already done so, to your realistic limits, and the price is still too high, then that is your problem (if you insist on staying open) or the consumer's problem (if he insists you stay open). The consumer may need financial help from his public trust (the government) but that is their battle. If the mental health center skips the consumer and looks to government for its financial input, then it is no longer dependent on the consumer. Its product is no longer measured against the most valid standard, the need of the consumer. If you do not care what the consumer needs or think you can create what he needs without giving him a chance to say "no thanks" then you are creating a giant myth machine, which will serve the idiosyncratic needs of those who choose to remain associated with it but not those *for whom* the machine was presumably built in the first place.

A careful distinction must be made here. When one looks at the medical resources available to people, and especially to poor people, two issues surface. They are often confused with each other. One has to do with the quality of the medical product, the quality of care being delivered. The second has to do with the delivery itself. The great attention being paid to delivery these days sometimes overlooks or makes certain assumptions about the quality of that which is to be delivered. There is something of a dilemma involved in attempting to solve the problems of quality of care and of delivery of service.

The assertion that funds should go from the consumer to the purveyor of service and *not* from governmental source to the purveyor is offered as a solution to the problem of *quality*. It gives the power of selection to the consumer, with the assumption that he will seek out quality and therefore reinforce it where it exists or stimulate it where it does not. The problem of delivery of health service is broader and is a public concern. As such it will require a heavier public hand, whether through fiscal policy or legislative regulation.

A mental health center may take on the task of developing sophisticated delivery systems and thereby be quite dependent on governmental funding. If it does so at the expense of quality of service, then it can "afford" to neglect the issue of the buying power of the consumer. A mental health center might wish to concentrate on quality of service rather than on the delivery systems but then fail to receive the proper consumer influence because so many consumers start out without any buying power. This is certainly the case in the urban centers where the mental health centers face enormous problems of poverty.

What happens too often is that the mental health center capitalizes on its governmental funding to expand and develop delivery systems and slides over the more delicately framed problem of quality of service.

Whether the buying power will eventually be provided through national insurance schemes or whether we will move towards pre-paid group service packages remains to be seen. It is important to realize that when the medical product is clear and unambiguous (surgical procedure, antimicrobial medication, etc.) then the feasibility of pre-paid group services is highest. The parameters of the product are distinct enough to make quality assessment possible. But in psychiatric services, the medical product is not so clear and so effectiveness might best be reinforced by allowing the consumer to exercise his buying power. He does not possess this if he is caught in the pre-paid service plan. In some ways this is similar to the catchment area closed market problem, but now clothed more clearly in economic trappings.

The problem becomes more complex when we realize that the probable costs of sophisticated delivery systems will exceed the money receivable from consumers regardless of how they, the consumers, get that money.

We are now faced with a dilemma. To program for quality services, the consumer should be our financial resource. But to deliver care (quality or not) we will need financial resources beyond the consumer. As we turn to the latter we undercut our means to a quality oriented service. Since the latter course is the one most prevalent in the community mental health movement, it is not surprising that quality of care is being relatively neglected.

This may seem a hornet's nest to the reader but I never promised to write an authenticated gospel.

chapter 5

CONTINUITY AND COMPREHENSIVE SERVICE:

Doing Everything Forever

Two of the key concepts in the community mental health movement are continuity of care and comprehensive care. These are basically problems in the delivery of health care and not problems relating to the nature of the care itself. Continuity suggests the delivery of health care *over time* as required by the idiosyncratic needs of the patient. It suggests a systematic monitoring of patient progress and the capacity to reinstitute medical care when it is required. Continuity of care is axiomatic to secondary and tertiary prevention since it suggests early intervention and maintenance of therapeutic gains.

Comprehensive care suggests the capacity to provide a wide range of services to correspond to the wide range of patient needs. It suggests the ability to coordinate different kinds of services so that a patient or family can avail themselves of the services without the common fragmentation or overlap.

Continuity and comprehensiveness are complementary and together provide a one-two punch towards improved delivery of health care. There are numerous confounding issues which could be considered. These are issues which speak to the mechanisms necessary to provide continuity and comprehensiveness of service, *e.g.* manpower types and distribution, generalized resources and specialized resources, reporting systems, outcome evaluation, sufficient funding and others. In this chapter we shall focus more directly on the concepts of specialization and generalization, welfare resources, and the concepts of continuity and comprehensiveness themselves. All of these concepts lend themselves to significant ambiguity and to unproductive idealism.

SPECIALIZED VS GENERALIZED APPROACH

There has been much debate about the necessity for specialization as against generalization in medical practice. Answers to this dilemma, as with answers to most dilemmas, come frequently from the heart rather than the brain. "Give me a good old-fashioned general practitioner" is the plaintive cry of the weary patient unable to find the specialist who can cure his multi-system hurt. "I have the best specialist in the East" is the proud claim of the patient with a broken leg, in cast, traction and elevation. It is a rare person who, at various times, cannot see the need for both the specialized *and* the generalized approach to problem solving.

A dilemma sets up two alternative positions which are mutually exclusive of each other. Both are enormously attractive and neither can be satisfactorily reasoned out of existence. So it is with the specialized vs generalized dichotomy. But the dilemma generates unnecessary confusion as well. It may be either/or for a specific problem at a specific time but it may be both for other problems at other times. Even general practitioners and specialists are learning to live with each other and occasionally succeed in working with each other. As with most dichotomous concepts, such as liberalism vs conservatism, activity vs passivity, good vs bad, and love vs hate, the two antagonists take turns on center stage. Wisdom and the lessons of history point out that the threat of excess by one antagonist is kept under constant check by the strength of the other. Too much liberalism is throttled by conservatism and vice versa.[1] From time to time one or the other seems clearly dominant but that is simply a pre-condition for the re-emergence of the other.

The same applies to the specialization vs generalization issue in medicine. Current assessment of the state of treatment orientations shows both approaches with strong backers although the specialists continue to proliferate at a greater rate than the generalists. The balance is maintained, however, by the tendency of specialists of different focus to organize themselves into more comprehensive group practices, *i.e.* more generalized units.

Specialization seems, in great measure, to follow the laws of supply and demand. As more and more information is accumulated the supply of information becomes greater than can be assimilated and utilized by solitary individuals. And so various individuals focus on various segments of the total available information and hence are called specialists. This puts highly differentiated skills into the hands of relatively few people. But differentiated skill is inversely proportional to generalized skill. If you know something about a lot of things, it is unlikely that you will also know a lot about a specific thing.

This natural antagonism between specialization and generalization is at the heart of the problem of discontinuous care afforded patients by our medical systems. The resolution of this tension in the interest of greater continuity will not come by specializing the generalist or by generalizing the specialist. It will come only when we have

1. An excellent overview of this dichotomous type of equilibrium, as seen in a broad historical perspective, can be found in Durant's *The Lessons of History* (New York: Simon and Schuster, 1968).

created a system of patient advocacy designed to fit the patient to the proper doses of specialization.

Specialized Resources

There are many ways of becoming specialized in one's work. Those who are knowledgeable and competent in the treatment of alcoholism, or schizophrenia, or geriatrics, or mental retardation, or drug abuse can be referred to as specialists. They are specialists in the treatment of generically grouped behavior. Those who are knowledgeable and competent in an emergency room, an out-patient department, a day-night hospital, or an in-patient department are generalists, *i.e.* they accept and attempt to treat people with various types of generic behavior. And yet isn't there a special skill attached to working in an emergency room or in an in-patient setting? Doesn't that make such persons specialists? What has happened is what inevitably happens when you try to concretize an abstraction. When you create a structure (like an emergency room) to concretize an abstraction, (like helping people in acute distress) you will inevitably become expert in the terms set down by your structure. Schizophrenics, and drug addicts, and seniles, and alcoholics, and mental retardates may come to your emergency room, each with certain generic differences, but the requirements of your structure (*i.e.* space, layout, personnel, politics, organization, administration, philosophy etc.) will give you a modus operandi especially suited to those structural requirements. In the process, persons with generically different needs will be served but the character of that service will be highly determined by the *special* resources and constraints of the structure.[2]

2. There is a deeper issue here, which is philosophic in quality and which cannot be dissected in this context. It is the intricate mutuality of the concepts of structure and function. Structure and function are abstractions from the synthesized, coordinated reality of our vital world. A structure functions and function structures. This intimate relationship is fundamentally a mutually-dependent one. There is no function without structure and no structure without function, just as there is no organism without context nor context without organism.

Those who are knowledgeable and competent in the treatment of children or adolescents can also be referred to as specialists. Here the discriminating feature is an age group rather than a specific pathologic feature of behavior. Implicit in this approach is the belief that there is information of such a quantity, and quality related to one age group or another, so as to necessitate a special expertise in their treatment.

Let us analyze the foregoing. Specialization seems to evolve around at least three orientations. There are specialists who focus on generic behavioral states; there are specialists who focus on treatment modalities; and there are specialists who focus on age clusters. When considered separately there is a seeming unproductive compartmentalizing. However, when considered together there is the germ of reason. The problem is that these various specialized resources are seldom seen together in one's thinking or in operation.

When a mental health center presents itself as an organization with emergency specialization, out-patient specialization, day-night hospital specialization, in-patient specialization and a variable mix of schizophrenic specialization, addiction specialization, alcoholic specialization, senility specialization, mental retardation specialization, children's problems specialization and adolescent problems specialization—it is guilty of unproductive compartmentalizing. But how does one pay necessary attention to the above specialized areas and simultaneously maintain a balance with a generalized view?

Generalized Resources

The extreme generalist would say "people with emotional distress are more alike than unlike. We can therefore treat people who the specialists would call alcoholics, addicts, schizophrenics, neurotics, retardates or what have you, with generally the same approach, given certain modifications here or there."[3] The specialist might smile at this and note that the modifications would be enormous. But anyone with more than passing experience with patients showing diverse behavioral phenomena should recognize that human beings do in fact show great similarities in their behavioral repertoire regardless of their individuality. Anxiety, depression, anger, fear, rationalization, intellectualization, motor activity, and other behavioral phenomena replicate themselves in different people experiencing different life circumstances. Isn't the administering of a tranquilizer for the anxiety of alcoholism, or of psychosis, or of neurosis, or of addiction, a testimony to the ubiquitous nature of that symptom?

The generalist position is intrinsically dependent on an abstracted view of man. He must extract from his patient those characteristics shared by all men and so he becomes expert in the commonality of men. The specialist is expert in the idiosyncracies of men. The generalist must take a patient as he is, avoiding to a large extent the special peculiarities. The specialist must take only those patients where he, the specialist, is expert. The specialist excludes first, while the generalist includes first.

Now then to the unanswered question: how does one pay necessary attention to the specialized areas and simultaneously maintain a balance with a generalization view? The answer is dependent on who is doing the answering and why. Implicit in the question is concern on a grand scale. It suggests that the question springs from someone concerned about the health needs of many people with

3. Psychiatric residency training follows this implicit rule more often than not, since it is based on an understanding of psychological processes which presumably all men share, rather than a focus on diseases which would emphasize idiosyncratic and discontinuous psychologic processes. The result is a putative homogenization of psychiatrists, making of them generalists in the treatment of psychologic disturbances—*rather than* specialists in the treatment of this group of disorders or that group of disorders.

diverse problems. It is implicitly a question which deals with a comprehensive orientation. It is not a question being asked by a surgeon. It is not a question being asked by a psychoanalyst. It is not a question being asked by a general practitioner. It is a question being asked by an advocate of patients. It is a question being asked by someone who wants the best of the generalist and the specialist for the sake of the patient. It is a question all patients should be asking but cannot because of the conceptual complexities.[4]

What I am suggesting is a third dimension, which we can term a patient advocacy system, analogous to the computer programmer. The programmer knows enough about the working of the computer to be able to give it certain general rules. The programmer in a real sense sets priorities and limits to the functioning of the computer. But he does not interfere with a specific computer function once that function has been activated. So too a patient advocacy system must have overall programming responsibility and the capacity to coordinate the functions of the various special and general resources at its command. This is a task requiring a great deal of sophistication, requiring working knowledge of the various specialized programs, the capacity for monitoring the progress of the patient and the capacity for activating or deactivating various special or general functions for specific patient problems.

When this patient flow is left to the idiosyncracies of separate specialized units, efficiency, consistency, effectiveness, comprehensiveness, and continuity all suffer. This

4. The advocate concept seems to emerge inevitably whenever there is a situation of great complexity wherein persons of less sophistication are unable equitably to pursue their own needs. Hence the lawyer represents us in the bewildering maze of jurisprudence. The medical system is being recognized as equally bewildering and so the idea of sophisticated advocates is emerging. The growing use of the ombudsman in other systems, (i.e. governments, universities, etc.) is a parallel development.

has been the style in the past and is the predominant style today, even in the innovative mental health centers.[5]

Expanding Horizons: The Social Welfare Resources

The preceding section gives an orientation which has validity not only for patient flow within the parent organization but for patient flow to other collaborative institutions or agencies as well. Most of the health and welfare agencies that are thought of as potential resources within the mental health net are characteristically specialized in their functions. They can provide service for this part or that part much as a surgeon will restrict his procedure. Beyond that the patient or client is on his own in the ubiquitous, confusing transfer-referral game.

There is great difficulty in incorporating disparate institutions, with varying goals, priorities, methods, philosophies, administrations, loyalties, etc. into a coherent caretaking system. Some have a public orientation while others are private. To hope for enlightened cooperative activity is as futile as hoping for a reconciliation between the mongoose and the snake. Self interest is not always consistent with public health interests. The alternatives are neither attractive nor feasible. On the one hand a center might try to develop all of the specialized functions within its own organization.[6] This will often lead to redundancy, but more realistically, would require the generation of new money and new personnel, neither of which can be readily

5. Medicine has carried within its marrow the very important quality of authoritativeness. Doctors have had to have the last word since patient responsibility has always ultimately resided with them. This has prepared doctors to be relatively autonomous and poor system men.

6. It is one of the magnificent peculiarities of governmental bureaucracy which establishes unrealistic goals as a matter of course. The mandate that community mental health centers should treat all of the various psychopathologies known to man from womb to tomb has been instrumental in developing a new jargon of comprehensiveness but not a new reality.

achieved. On the other hand, the coordinated and comprehensive cooperation between agencies could be forced by the withholding of public funds from those agencies that would not negotiate their autonomy for the larger program. Here the risk of centralized mediocrity looms large because of the tradition of governmental mediocrity in the health and welfare domain. At any rate both of these alternatives exist and there are probably more. To pursue them further at this point would unduly fatigue both the author and the reader.

The Problem of Coordinating Linkage

The heart of this chapter thus far has been in its argument for a so-called patient advocacy system as a coordinating and patient programming operation. There are certain aspects of this system that deserve further elaboration. These can perhaps be best considered under the rubrics of quality control and quantity control.

Quality Control

Quality is a slippery concept. One man's quality may be another man's poison. It is connotative more than it is denotative. But to deal with such a concept in an operational context it must be made denotative. Any operational function can be examined at the level of goals, methods and outcome. If goals and methods are made explicit, then one could determine to what extent the methods led to an outcome consistent with the goals. An operation which is marked by a congruence of goals and outcome can be considered a quality operation. It accomplished what it set out to accomplish. The methods then meet the quality standard as made explicit in the goals.

But the methods may also have to meet quality standards derived not from the goals but from other value systems considered relevant. For example, if a quality outcome occurred in a method system that was basically dehumanizing it would be hard to call the method a quality method. Consider a young man, acutely psychotic and excited. The therapeutic goal might be to reduce the psychotic symptoms and excitement but if this were accomplished with failure to reassure family, locking the patient in a filthy cramped room and failing to provide basic personal amenities, then the method could hardly be characterized as showing quality. Quality therefore must be measured not only against goal and outcome congruence, but against explicit standards of care as well.

One further dimension is necessary in this quality system. It is important to recognize at the outset that the statement of goals must reflect the combined wisdom of the patient advocate system and the *patient himself*. It may very easily develop that the goals established for any given patient will be a compromise between the original

QUALITY CONTROL

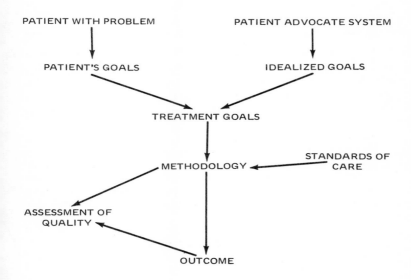

goal outline of the advocate and the original goal intent of the patient. But to be able to ultimately say something about quality of care one must first bring in the patient's own goals for seeking help.[7]

Quantity Control

Quantity ultimately boils down to numbers. Numbers of patients, numbers of personnel, numbers of man hours, numbers of dollars, etc. In the quantity control function of the patient advocacy system primary attention needs to be paid to the cost per unit of service (however defined). This unit cost must then be judged against the outcome measures (cost-benefit analysis). How much is it costing, in this case, to get these specific outcomes. Or, more embarrassingly, how much is it costing, in this case, to get a poor quality outcome. Until this type of cost accounting becomes an integral facet of a total treatment organization, there will be no way of judging the ultimate value of the organization in the very important economic world of reality.

In many ways the patient advocacy system is at the heart of the delivery of care system. It is a programming and calibrating system with very definite cybernetic implications. It cannot work without explicit directions, much as a computer programmer cannot work without being very explicit. It means forms and lists and check-

7. This is a controversial point of view. A mainstay of traditional psychoanalytic therapy has been the idea that the doctor knows best and so the patient's complaint must await the development of the therapeutic process. He might have to eventually be shown that his original complaint was incidental, irrelevant or a camouflage for the real problem. Such an attitude can confound legitimate attempts to measure outcome, but more importantly, it tends to belittle the patient's more immediate access to his inner world, in favor of the therapist's more limited and more theoretical access to that world.

marks and machines. It means responsibility and prerogatives. It means organizational technology.[8]

CONTINUITY

At the heart of continuity is the concept of time. One cannot hope to understand continuity if one does not first understand time. At first glance this seems much ado about nothing, but it is quite the opposite. When we begin to talk about a *plan over time* we do so *in time*. That is we talk *today* about something which is to happen tomorrow. Our awareness of tomorrow (as we consider it today) is limited by what is available to us today. If an architect plans a building, he does so with the knowledge that his plan is being created from To to Tn but his building is being created from Tn to Tn + x. During that duration of time, from Tn to Tn + x, a multiplicity of unforeseen events may occur necessitating certain modifications of the original plan. The original plan is, as possible, a close approximation to the real process of building the building but an approximation nonetheless. What makes the building a reality is the capacity of architect and builders to respond to the unforeseen events and adjust the plan accordingly.

The same principle obtains, but with great precision, in the workings of a thermostatically controlled furnace. The functioning of the furnace *depends* on the feedback available to it via the thermostat. No one could hope to program the furnace at the time of installation so that it could provide heat at a stable level over time. No one can predict what the climatic temperature variations will be from day to day.

8. Organizational technology means more than administrative expertise. It presumes an articulated understanding not only at the product end, *i.e.* the dimensions of care and its delivery system, but also of the nature of systems, groups and other organizational units.

This is perhaps an over-elaborate way of stating that a system, which insures continuity of care, depends on the cybernetic principle. It means that there must be *at any point in time*, a set of patient *conditions* which, when reported to the medical system, *triggers* an *appropriate system function*. In that concise statement are many patches of quicksand. It is one thing to logically construct a continuity system on paper, but a vastly different thing to get one to work with more than primitive efficiency.

Consider first the *patient conditions* that indicate care is needed. This is a statement which presumes objective clarity. It presumes that there *are* specific conditions of health or disease that correspond to the need or non-need for health care. A case can certainly be made for the position that there are numerous rather clear-cut objective indices that should precipitate health care. These are most clear in the "harder" medical specialties where signs are often as prevalent as symptoms. But in the psychiatric field signs are less prevalent than symptoms. Much of the patient condition is a *subjective* phenomenon. To be sure, there are numerous objective signs of mental disorder but these are generally of the type which require certain investigative sophistication. For example, dissociation may not be noted if there is no careful mental status examination. Delusions may not be noted if there is no conversation. Hallucinations may not be noted if the patient does not offer the evidence. And these are the more gross of the objectifiable psychiatric signs.

The reality is that for much of psychiatric morbidity, the phenomena are beyond the awareness of the environment. Their disclosure is very often a function of the patient's *desire* to disclose. This leads to a very important point. Psychotic behavior may be as much of the terrain of morbidity that we can reasonably hope to incorporate into a system for continuity of care. And even in the case of psychotic behavior we will only be able to pick up that behavior which is objectifiable and identifiable.

This problem of *covert patient condition* casts a long shadow over the wish to create effective systems for continuity of care. If the system depends on the willingness of the patient to *report* his subjective state to the system, then the system is only as good as the willingness of the patient to report. That is precisely where we have been right along and so this is hardly a step towards the solution of the problem of better continuity of care.

This patient inertia (towards a reluctance to report subjective phenomena) is quite general, in that it can be seen in all types of behavior, and in all types of people. There are probably certain class related predispositions as well. Lower classes seem less prone to divulge subjective states or, when disposed to do so, are less able to effectively communicate that state.[9]

The net effect of all of this is to conclude that the continuity system cannot be built on patient motivation. The alternative is a system which employs periodic surveying of all known cases. This enormously expensive approach, which has been Madison Avenued by the term "reaching out,"[10] is only as good as the survey instrument on the one hand and its practicality as a repeatable operation on the other. This is often a recycling case-finding survey. There are numerous survey instruments that can identify various behavior states but these have generally been used to answer questions of incidence or prevalence. That is a vastly different use than the periodic use and re-use to assess fluctuations in the development of behavior states (that is the problem in continuity systems).

9. Bernstein, B.: Social Class, Speech Systems, and Psychotherapy, *British Journal of Sociology*, March 1964.
10. "Reaching out" is a phrase which covers a variety of operations but in general they all suggest an aggressive pursuit of the patient, in contrast to the traditional waiting for the patient to come to the office. The "reaching out" concept has developed a connotative image reminiscent of Michelangelo's famous Sistine Chapel fresco showing the outstretched hand of God delivering life to the welcoming hand of Adam.

But even if we were able to develop practical instruments (or standardized follow-up interviews) other problems await us.

A stimulus without a response is like kissing the air. If the patient's condition warrants intervention and if it is detected and if it is reported, then the medical system had better respond. The maintenance of an efficient detection and reporting phase depends on the maintenance of a responding medical system. This is true in the first place because of the reinforcement afforded the survey reporters by seeing their work pay off. It is important beyond that because the expense incurred in reaching out is not justifiable unless there is medical response and reasonable achievement of secondary or tertiary prevention. Presumably we are willing to incur the initial expenses of aggressive monitoring because this will lead to greater economy in long-range patient care.

The troubles begin when the monitoring becomes efficient. No one is quite sure about what would be required to provide competent long-range care *as well as* competent short-range care. We seem reasonably proficient at short-term efforts but also seem sufficiently busy. How busy we would be by enlarging the case-load remains to be seen. The argument, of course, is that eventually we will be seeing fewer relapses because of our more careful follow-up and maintenance regimens. The fact of fewer relapses presumes greater economy of man hours by care-giving staff but the whole rationale is built with theoretical benediction.

It is impossible to argue very convincingly against the concept of continuity. It is clear that the natural history of many diseases is marked by disappearance and reappearance and that medical needs therefore must be responded to over time. Thus far continuity has been best provided in those circumstances where initiative for maintaining continuity has *come from* the patient himself. His own desire to receive help when he perceived its need has been the guarantor of continuity where it has occurred. Now we are considering ways of insuring continuity with the initiative coming from the medical resource rather than the patient. As difficult as this will be for most medical problems it will be most difficult in those conditions generally regarded as psychiatric problems.

The corollary to these conclusions is ominous. In the psychiatric field, attempts to insure continuity (as initiated by the medical resource) will require a degree of mechanization and intrusion into the lives of others that may be abhorent. And even at that, the likelihood that a system (initiated by the resource) will adequately speak to the needs of continuity is questionable. When all the tinkering with the machine is over, the only model that has a reasonable chance of surviving is a mutual need model. If a condition exists where there is simultaneous incentive in the resource *and* the consumer, which prompts them to reach out to each other, then we will see adequate continuity. To achieve this, two conditions must exist: the *quality* of care being provided by a medical resource must be sufficiently obvious to attract those who have need and the consumer must have the *buying power* to choose his service resource. Under those conditions the resource will depend on attracting consumers for its existence and the consumer will be stimulated to initiate continuity of care by the attraction of quality service.

COMPREHENSIVENESS

The recognition that there is a need for comprehensive care comes at a time when fragmentation of services is at its highest. The ever continuous development of specialists will not stop. It is a natural and necessary condition of rapidly expanding knowledge and information. The problem now is the coordination of the multiple specialized parts of the whole health delivery package.

There are two distinct problems that should be differentiated at the outset. One is the problem of coordination which generated our earlier discussion of a patient advocacy system. The other has to do with the concept of comprehensiveness itself. It is this latter issue which will be the focus of this section.

Comprehensiveness is a concept that has meaning along a continuum. The problems that humans face are a necessary part of their humanness. They come as part of the evolutionary challenge. Adapt or die is the ultimate rule. The varieties of challenge and the quantifiable differences in these challenges that every human faces are beyond our mathematical cognition. The process of living one's life is the unfolding of challenge and response. It varies enormously from individual to individual. And what follows, necessarily and logically, is that the "need for service" varies enormously from individual to individual.

Society has been looking at the "needs" of individuals since Sumer and has been developing institutions to serve *some* of these needs ever since. The kinds of helping institutions that have been developed have varied according to the availability of knowledge and resource to do a job. They have also depended on the collective will to create such institutions (public responsibility) or on entrepreneurial initiative (private enterprise). The ultimate in comprehensiveness suggests the availability of an institution for every imaginable problem. This is possible only in the imagination and will never be a reality. Collective man is forever moving back and forth between the status quo and the promise over the horizon. That concern for "progress" has a higher priority than helping the individual casualties who, for whatever reason, cannot maintain an adaptive viability. If there are enough individual casualties of one sort or another, then society generates an institution to care for them (more or less), in direct proportion to the ability of the casualties to demand help.[11]

11. It is important to learn the lesson of the squeaking wheel. The very old and the very young, the mentally ill, the imprisoned and the retarded all share an inability to demand society's attention. The quality and quantity of humane care available for

And so total comprehensiveness of care is in some ways contrary to our collective nature. That is one dimension of the limits on comprehensiveness. Another limit comes from the ubiquitous meaning of the term itself. How much care is enough to qualify as comprehensive? If a man has heart disease, diabetes, gout, depression and anxiety, does he need care for them all? Does he want care for them all? Is care available for them all? If he is also unemployed, living in over-crowded quarters, and unsophisticated in the ways of the surrounding culture, does he need care for any or all of them? Does he want care for them? Is care available? The following laws are certain. It is possible to think of more problems than it is to think of answers. It is possible to think of more answers than it is to act them out. It is possible to act out more answers than it is to have them work.

Comprehensiveness is like an itch. The more you scratch, the more you itch. The ultimate comprehensiveness is an infantilizing dream. Between the present and the dream there is still much left to be desired. But what should guide us in searching for a realistic concept of comprehensive care? The traditional limits of medicine have helped in establishing what most people mean by comprehensive health care. But Public Health and psychiatry have, historically pushed those limits further and now community psychiatry has made a shambles of the boundary lines. The implication can be stated in a question. Why shouldn't comprehensive health care include care of social problems that inevitably influence health, like poverty, overcrowding and poor education? This is where we enter a thicket full of thorns and seductive berries.

Let us make another distinction before proceeding. When thought of in medical terms, comprehensiveness sug-

---

them should suggest that society does not often respond without being driven by significant numbers of franchised members. The above, silent groups have lost their franchise, their voice, their power but not their right to helpful care.

gests the coordinated provision of health services. We shall refer to this as a comprehensive health services package. When thought of with a community psychiatry orientation it suggests the provision of health and more general welfare services. We shall refer to this as a broad-spectrum comprehensive services package.

Those who are neither short-sighted nor narrow-minded immediately sense that comprehensive care could and should include not only those more traditional medical services, but at least those established social services (including legal, education and general welfare) that are already available in society but outside the health care field. The packaging of all these services in a more comprehensive wrapping is delectable to the comprehensive health planner. So much for the berries.

The thorns come from the medical ethos itself. Not the ethos of the reactionary physician content to do his particular specialty and that alone. Not the conservative ethos, dramatically caricatured by medical organizations such as the American Medical Association. The thorns come from the very persons who grandly accept the relevance of extending the health care package so as to make of it a broad-spectrum comprehensive services package. The thorns are a function of the power acquisitiveness of the comprehensive health planner. The very openness, boldness and ingenuity which fed his leadership in the planning, will feed his oligarchic needs in the operation. The broad-spectrum comprehensive services package, if born of medical parents, will forever bear their resemblance.

In many ways, it is understandable that medicine, and particularly social and/or community psychiatry, is intrigued with developing ever more comprehensive programs. Other professionals in the social sciences, have been more interested in studying problems than in mounting programs of intervention. And when they have developed programs, they have generally kept them discrete and unidimensional, not comprehensive and multidimensional.

Besides this "filling a vacuum" effect there are other reasons for medical leadership in the comprehensive planning business.

The medical industry is one of the largest industries in America, and as such is enormously powerful. It is within the nature of the powerful to gravitate towards new power. It is therefore quite natural for medicine to see itself as the centerpiece in the broad-spectrum comprehensive care package. Secondly, the physician has a tradition of willingness to assume responsibility. Having started with the enormous responsibilities inherent in the treatment of many life and death conditions in his patients, it is a short illusory jump to the responsibility for social malaise.

The reader may be holding his head in despair at this point. How can the conservative, narrow, entrepreneur who is a physician, be described as bold and eager to lead? It is tempting but wrong to generalize excessively as a ten-year-old lemming might gleefully inform us. Although the medical establishment is basically conservative it has notable exceptions. These exceptions are to be found outside the medical laboratories and surgical suites. These exceptions are administrative-politico types or community-clinician types and their numbers swell yearly. And the fact that they are still solidly identified with the medical profession attaches great power and prestige to their efforts.

But the point has not been adequately made. Why is the medical leadership of a broad-spectrum comprehensive services package less than the best? Why is medical leadership a thorn in the thicket? To answer this adequately is to take yet another side road.

In the earlier reference to the various and multiple problems which can be identified as indigenous to being a human, we failed to discuss the concepts of priority and resource as they attach to these various problems. If the Sumerians were faced with extinction by a nomadic tribe at their borders, and by a plague within their borders, they would have probably created an army. Their resources were better suited to waging war than to eradicating disease. If a doctor is faced with a patient suffering from congestive heart failure and chronic sinusitis he will probably treat the heart condition first. The priority is clear. At the core of priority rests the fact that you can't always do everything and you may have to *choose* among many possibilities. At the core of resource rests the fact that you may not be able to do something (even if the top priority) if you don't have the where-with-all to do it. Resource and priority are at the bedrock of effective work.

When we now turn to the issue of broad-spectrum comprehensive service we can start by noting the multiplicity of problems that can be faced. When a doctor looks at the problem of comprehensive service he sees medical needs first and then the extension into the many socio-economic and legal-political ramifications. He sees a health care package with extensions into the social context. A doctor is likely to have medical priorities as well as knowledge about the availability of medical resources. The point is that the broad-spectrum comprehensive services package, led by a physician, will be a comprehensive health package with medical expertise and medical resources. The status of "comprehensiveness" *beyond* the medical borders (*e.g.* legal services, social work services, employment and rehabilitation services, education and welfare services) will be ultimately of secondary stature. From a medical point of view this is reasonable and proper. But what then happens is that these other non-medical services fail to develop and coordinate themselves to the degree required by the needs of people. By the marginal inclusion of "social services" in the comprehensive health package, a sort of tokenism will have been accomplished and their domination by medicine will have been perpetuated.

This may seem an unnecessary diversion to the reader, especially in view of the enormous need now apparent in medicine for a radical restructuring, reordering of priorities, and development of better medical delivery systems. To the extent that comprehensive health planning remains focused on fairly traditional health services, then I would concur with such efforts. My objection rests with the tendency to extrapolate that comprehensive health plan (probably through the conduit of community mental health) to include social, legal and economic services. It is because these latter are so critically necessary that I would object to their being short-changed by inclusion into and under a medical plan.

The message is really rather simple. If, by comprehensive, we consider a wide range of problems that go beyond the borders of medical care, then the comprehensive planning and control should not rest within medicine. If, by comprehensive, we consider the range of variations within medicine itself, then obviously its planning and control should remain within medicine. If one looks to the horizon one will not see any promising activity in the direction of development of broad-spectrum comprehensive services. Comprehensive medical planning yes, but broader planning no, except in those instances where it is "talked about" within the medical plan.

There are only two institutions, massive enough and expert enough, which could mount the beginning models of a broad-spectrum comprehensive services plan. These are the federal government and the university. Neither could do it alone but together it would be possible. In such a scheme, medicine (including psychiatry) would be a *part* and not the whole. In this scheme the priority of health services could be measured against the priority of the other welfare services and overall coordination of the entire broad-spectrum comprehensive service package would rest outside of medicine.

PATIENT FREEDOM AND CONFIDENTIALLY

Whenever men sit down to construct systems, an inevitable process occurs. The parts of the systems (whether they be inanimate or living) begin to lose their intrinsic unpredictability. A system is only as good as its predictability and so all of the parts must be forced into the patterns and programs of the system. When we talk about systems to provide continuity and comprehensiveness, we are invariably talking about people. There are those people who work within the system (producers) and those people for whom the system is ultimately constructed (consumers). Because they are people and because people have a built-in system jamming apparatus, the best laid plans may go awry. A human system is only an approximation and subject to the most extraordinary contradictory impulses of people. But a dedicated system builder will join the fray with zest. The unpredictable nature of producers and consumers is just another challenge to his ingenuity. It calls for system tightening, greater reliance on non-human technologic mechanisms and freedom reducing legislation "for the good of the consumer." Home visiting teams may ultimately give way to job visiting teams. Psychotherapy in the office has already moved to the living room and kitchen and may soon be in the bedroom. Three consecutive missed appointments may no longer call for termination but rather a "reaching out" onslaught on the home. A subpoena of the doctor's records may become a subpoena of the central computer's tapes.

But the dilemma rests with the fact that in the provision of service, with a condition of excessive demand and limited supply, only efficient distribution systems (with centralized planning and control) will suffice. If there were greater service resources, the need for centralization might be less. There is an iron-clad relationship between freedom and socialism. The greater the degree of individual freedom the greater will be the mal-distribution of goods and services. When the mal-distribution is sufficient to enrage the poor, a swing towards social control ensures. This social centrism limits individual freedom and, when this limiting is sufficient to enrage the enslaved, a swing towards decentralization ensues.

At this moment in history we find ourselves in a situation of mal-distribution of goods and services. The solution, despite the variations on the theme that will emerge, will move us towards greater social control from above. When plugged into the medical and other human services systems that will mean less patient freedom and less confidentiality. That will be a price for tightening the system and correcting the mal-distribution.

Is the price too high for the product? The instinct says yes, since personal freedom is deep in our marrow. But the animals that climbed aboard Noah's Ark gave up much of their freedom in the interest of survival. The rule is invariable: when freedom threatens species survival, freedom declines.

The important question is not should we resist the encroachment on patient freedom and confidentiality BUT rather how can we ensure that the decrease of freedom is quantitatively and qualitatively controlled? The danger is not that there will be less freedom but rather that the degree of loss of freedom will be more than the system truly needs to be efficient. The problem is that we are dealing with pendulum swings and not micrometer settings. We may need to chop down some trees to provide enough wood for shelter but do we need to chop down the entire forest? It is a question of control of excess.

Since it is probably inevitable that error will be part of the solution, let us insist that we err in omission rather than in commission. Let each hunk of freedom be zealously guarded and give the system builder a minimal number of concessions. It is too easy to go too far too fast.

TOWARDS A SUPERMARKET MODEL

The comprehensive services model, whether we refer to medical or broad-spectrum comprehensiveness, has many potential prototypes in our open-marketplace. The corporate retail institutions which sell multiple products under one roof have brought quality and efficiency with reduced consumer cost. The supermarket model used in the grocery industry, or in the "department store" industry, is worth our consideration as a model for the comprehensive services.

There are two characteristics of the supermarket that are particularly relevant. Before a supermarket decides on a location it surveys an area to determine its potential in terms of consumers and in convenience of access. If there are enough people in that area who could be predicted to be consumers and if the location is convenient for the consumer, then the supermarket may be placed there. The second characteristic of the supermarket is its attention to the quality and price of its products. If, through efficiency and proper management, it can provide greater quality or lower price (or both) then it is competitive and viable. The benefactors will be both the consumer people and the service people.

The area around a supermarket will usually provide the bulk of consumers. It does so because of convenience for the consumer. But a consumer is free to travel to any other supermarket if for reasons of quality or price he so chooses. There is no catchment area to entrap the consumer.

Once in a supermarket the consumer can easily get to the products he needs with a minimum of confusion. If he cannot find the department that handles his needed product, he can easily be informed and properly directed, rapidly and conveniently. He won't be required to travel across the city for eggs and back again for meat.

If, instead of a supermarket, we were talking about a comprehensive service center, very little of the above would have to be changed. The building might look different, the service employees would have different products, the consumer would have different needs, but the essential ingredients (service resource, consumer need, quality and cost of product, and open-market economy) would prevail.

In some ways community psychiatry, in its primitive community mental health center structure, is a vanguard operation for an ultimate supermarket model of comprehensive service. If it could see this long range perspective, some of its current malaise might be easier to tolerate. The missing link, however, is the sponsor or convener of the various services within the comprehensive service center. We have already warned of the dangers inherent in medical sponsorship and have indicated a preference for a tandem governmental-university sponsorship of the pilot program. How long it will take and where it will occur are questions that only time will answer.

chapter 6

PREVENTION:

Today's Burp Is Tomorrow's Ulcer

The ultimate exercise in man's omnipotent view of himself is his preoccupation with controlling the future. "The war to end all wars" was the credo of prevention several wars ago. History is replete with massive efforts designed to prevent this or that. Invariably, the efforts themselves get swallowed in the hidden processes that shape history and what may start "as a prevention" is eventually "the cause of."

What emerges, as one reflects on man's efforts to prevent future events from occurring, is the general rule that prevention is directly proportional to the control of causative variables. What follows, on a practical level rather than as an absolute, is that the greater the number of causative variables for an event, the less likely is the prospect of "preventing" that event. When dealing with an event having multiple causative variables, efforts to control those variables must be successful if prevention is to succeed. Partial success at control does not prevent, it merely modifies the event and more often than not it does so *in an unpredictable manner.*

The implication of the above is that most efforts at prevention of future behavioral events really tend to modify the events in an unpredictable fashion. This seemingly cynical cornerstone plays itself out in community psychiatry over and over again.[1] The nature of the problems dealt with by psychiatry are inherently frustrating and their intractable nature tends to undermine the need for an effective identity for the psychiatrist. The kind of work that goes on between patient and therapist is laborious and progress is measured in millimeters. It is no wonder that the yearning for prevention runs deeply.

THE PREVENTION OF PREVENTION

If it is true that most efforts at prevention turn out to be causative agents of unpredictable events then we can consider the consequences of such action. It seems almost sinful to proceed with this basic assumption because the concept of prevention is so dear to all of us. Perhaps the burden can be lightened somewhat by recalling that prevention is in fact feasible, effective (and even noble) in many instances where the undesirable event is prevented by successful control of the relatively *few* causative variables involved. This is most obvious in medicine in the progress made in immunology, sanitation, certain surgical

1. Within the Temple University Community Mental Health Center voices were constantly raised, from all disciplines, professional and non-professional alike, declaring the need to "get to the cause of mental illness" by dealing with the social problems rampant in the catchment area. As an example the following is a stated purpose of one of several competing community boards attempting to influence mental health center policy: "to resolve the underlying causes of mental health problems such as unequal distribution of opportunity, income, and benefits of technical progress."

procedures, antimicrobial procedures, and wherever a villain has been clearly identified. The thrust of this discussion, however, has to do with a quality of event, human behavior, that is so ubiquitous and multi-determined, that its causality and hence its predictability is grossly obscure.

The vocabulary says prevention but the intervention is less a prevention than it is a new cause. Since the object of prevention is usually an "undesirable," we might reasonably call our efforts benevolent gambling. We hope the end result will show at least some diminution of the undesirable phenomena, but it very well may bear no resemblance to our intent. And this is where the justification for preventive programming must be established. Does the preventer have sufficient knowledge of the essential causal variables *and* does he have sufficient control over them? If the answer to either of these questions is no, then call it benevolent gambling and not prevention.

In today's community mental health game many have become intrigued with the findings, like those of Hollingshead and Redlich,[2] which describe a direct relationship between social class and mental illness.[3] A relationship does not always mean a causative relationship as most would agree. Despite this, however, it is still common to hear vocal and militant voices shouting for a prevention of mental illness through an attack on the social conditions which *cause* them. To claim that social conditions should not be changed would be absurd in the face of our very

2. Hollingshead, A. B. and Redlich, F. C.: *Social Class and Mental Illness*. New York: Wiley, 1958.
3. In Hollingshead and Redlich, op. cit, 1958, they offer, to this point: "In our search for the etiological components of disorders, we would like to know the stresses and presses, as well as the conflicts, the rewards, and punishments of primary and secondary groups, particularly as far as they are related to social class. While our data indicate that sociocultural factors are important in the prevalence of treated disorders in the population, we cannot conclude they are the essential and necessary conditions in the etiology of mental disorders." p.360.

visible social malaise, but to suggest that these changes will invariably prevent mental illness is equally absurd.[4/5/6/7] If a mental health center wishes to embark on that course let it do so but let it identify what it is it wishes to do: benevolent gambling and *not* prevention.

DETERMINISM AND THE PUMP HANDLE

The paradigm of successful prevention has been the act of Snow, who removed the pump handle from the town's well after discovering that the contaminated water was the cause of cholera among the townsfolk.[8] That is a good example of linear causality: A causes B. The isolation of the viral villain in the causation of poliomyelitis led eventually to its control and hence to its prevention. That is also a good example of linear causality. But the multiple events and phenomena of the world are not all parts of linear causal chains. Most events are like icebergs, with a small visible and understood area but a vast invisible and unknown causal matrix. This diffuse interconnecting causal network is further complicated by multiple time-bound inputs and by the weight of prior events back through history to "earth's first clay." We are at a level of understanding of most human events which rivals the level of cosmic understanding enjoyed by the amoeba. Despite

4. French, J. R. P., Jr.: The Social Environment and Mental Health. *Journal of Social Issues*, 19, 39–56, 1963.
5. Fried, M.: Social Problems and Psychopathology, in Group for the Advancement of Psychiatry (Ed.), *Urban American and the Planning of Mental Health Services*, Washington, D.C., 1964, pp. 403–446.
6. Fried, M., and Lindemann, E.: Sociocultural Factors in Mental Health and Illness, *American Journal of Orthopsychiatry*, 31, 87–101, 1961.
7. Greenblatt, M., Emery, P. E. and Glueck, B. C.: *Poverty and Mental Health*. Washington, D.C.: American Psychiatric Association, 1967.
8. Snow, J.: *Snow on Cholera*, New York: The Commonwealth Fund, 1936.

our protestations and arrogant confidence we are lived more than we live.

When we in psychiatry wave our preventive banners, we must look ridiculous to even the gods on Mount Olympus who once held the key to the causal mysteries of human events. But surely between the pump handle and the primordial beginning there must be a rational place for the preventive psychiatrist.

The concepts of primary, secondary and tertiary prevention provide us with a way out of the mess, and allow us the continued use of the coveted term, prevention. We will not define these concepts here since they are so well standardized and publicized as public health commandments. Suffice to say that primary prevention suggests total obliteration of the villain so that no sign of his villainous deed can be found. Secondary prevention suggests that the undesirable event (illness) has occurred and the task is now to obliterate it (the illness not the causal villain) and "prevent" it from occurring again if possible. Tertiary prevention suggests that the undesirable event is now with us to stay (chronic illness) and the task is to "prevent" it from progressing to an even more undesirable situation. Each degree from primary through tertiary suggests a compromise and an attempt to reduce the odds which work towards adaptive decompensation.[9/10] There is also a sense of logical progression from primary to secondary to tertiary which is seductive in its clarity and erroneous in its connotation. The gap, conceptually and operationally, between primary prevention and secondary prevention is enormous. The great bulk of our information, experience, and theorizing has been focused on issues of secondary and

9. Berger, D. G., Rice, C. E., Sewall, L. G. and Lemkau, P. V.: The Impact of Psychiatric Hospital Experience On the Community Adjustment of Patients, *Mental Hygiene*, 49, 83–93, 1965.
10. Roen, S. R., Ottenstein, D., Cooper, S. and Burnes, A.: Community Adaptation As An Evaluative Concept in Community Mental Health, *Archives of General Psychiatry*, 15, 36–44, 1966.

tertiary prevention. We limp along in that pursuit but we at least have some sense of the dimensions. In the primary prevention of selected human behavior we have little information, little experience and some theory.[11] The role of the preventive psychiatrist then should be one which leads to the generation of new information, experience and theory. The preventive psychiatrist, in short, is engaged in research and his activities should be clearly identified as such.[12]

THE UBIQUITOUS CHILD AND HIS SHAPING

Preventive programs have a way of becoming child oriented.[13/14/15] They come from our sense of historical determinism which led Wordsworth to say that "The child is father of the man." If what happened yesterday is somehow the reason for what happened today, then logic suggests we deal with the yesterdays. That process has its final logical target in the child since he is today's yesterday and since, in his relative helplessness, he is so much more manipulable. Children are pushed, pulled, led, trained, reinforced, punished, rewarded, warned, educated and brainwashed by the collaborative conspiracy of parents and society. Our vision is that if we could "raise" a child *properly* we would have a splendid and normal adult, much as well-leavened dough becomes fat bread. And so the preventively oriented psychiatrist would like to get

11. Caplan, G.: *Principles of Preventive Psychiatry*. New York: Basic Books, 1964.
12. Research, in its most fundamental sense, is the handmaiden of prevention. It attempts to isolate causal variables and give direction to the control of these variables.
13. Schiff, S. K., and Kellam, S. G.: A Community-wide Mental Health Program of Prevention and Treatment in First Grade, *Psychiatric Research Report American Psychiatric Association*, 21:92, 1967.
14. Stickney, S. B.: Schools Are Our Community Mental Health Centers, *American Journal Psychiatry*, 124:1407, 1968.
15. Kaplan, G. (Ed.): *Prevention of Mental Disorders in Children*. New York: Basic Books, 1961.

into that kitchen. More often than not, he settles for the school and its handle on child rearing.

True to the principle of reductio ad absurdum, however, many have discovered that even the school years are too late and so on to Head Start and Get Set.[16] It won't be long before we follow the trail to the delivery room or to the wedding bed. The point is that the preventive psychiatrist has a glimpse of part of that submerged iceberg and is following it as though it were the whole iceberg. Certainly that part of the iceberg is tremendously important and we know child-rearing practices play a role in what comes later. But to see child rearing in the linear causal dimension is to miss its *partial* importance in the total causal matrix. This is not to say that working with children, whether at home or in the schools, will not help make them better at something or other but that is the point. It makes them better at something or other that has its causal variables out in the open and ready for control. Those gains may be significant but it is uncertain that the yield can be extrapolated to the multiple kinds of maladaptive states we witness in adulthood. There is no more compelling reason to expect that all the causal variables of adult pathology reside in childhood than there is to expect that all of them reside contemporaneously with adulthood.

THE TEMPTATION OF TAUTOLOGY

The causal variables of human behavior are rascals. They will not sit still long enough for us to measure them, there are more of them than we can handle and they appear and disappear in time. They sometimes travel in a straight line and sometimes in clusters. Some may be at home with anthropologists, while others are known by the sociologists. Others devil political scientists or economists. Some appear four times a week on an analyst's couch while yet others will only speak to a biophysicist. Together they

16. Richmond, J. B.: Communities in Action: A Report on Project Head Start, *Journal of Pediatrics*, 37:905, 1966.

have maintained a conspiracy against students of human behavior so as to render them *all* partially impotent. It may be part of the master plan to forever keep us far at bay. They may give us a glimpse of this or a piece of that but never the whole picture.

But with this humble perspective it would seem reasonable to expect much futility in the prevention business. Thus far this expectation has not been upset.[17] Prevention is always around the next corner or over the next horizon. The force which seems to perpetuate our optimism is our tendency to see human behavior as a more complicated but yet controllable phenomenon, as seen in the technological mastery over our environment. The examples in physics and the other hard sciences inspire us onward. But all of the victories in science which led to the ability to predict and therefore control are based on phenomena whose causal variables resided within one or few levels of organization. There are undoubtedly many human behaviors which also have their causal variables within one or few levels of organization. An example is the genetic research on the etiology of schizophrenia.[18] But so much of human behavior has origins in multiple levels of organization that we shall never achieve the kind of predictability and control that we see in the technologic sciences.[19]

But the die-hard will persist in his attempts and this is good since without the ultimate illusion we might not discover many of the helpful bits and pieces that come from

17. An excellent critique and overview of programs of primary prevention was given in a paper delivered to the forty-seventh annual meeting of the American Orthopsychiatric Association: Garmezy, N.: *Vulnerability Research and the Issue of Primary Prevention*, March, 1970.

18. Rosenthal, D., and Kety, S. S. (Editors): *The Transmission of Schizophrenia*, New York: Pergamon Press, 1968.

19. An excellent discussion of the complexity of behavioral determinism, from a general systems point of view, can be found in Anatol Rapoport's foreword in the sourcebook, *Modern Systems Research For the Behavioral Scientist*, Edited by Walter Buckley (Chicago: Aldine Publishing Company, 1968).

his researchs. The preventive psychiatrist is a bits and pieces practitioner with built-in chutzpa. He takes this piece and that, fills the gaps with maybe, packages his war on evil so that it will be funded and sets out. What he often discovers soon enough is that he has been dealing with a tautology right along. A tautology is a statement which attempts to explain everything and therefore explains nothing. It is a trick of nature perpetrated on our minds that we cannot begin to explain the grand scale phenomena without losing sight of the small scale phenomena. And likewise we cannot explain the small scale phenomena without losing sight of the grand scale phenomena. The grand scale and the small scale are not inconsistent with each other but we can't deal with them both at the same time.

There is a growing awareness that the causative variables of human behavior are so vast and elusive that no one discipline or even confederation of several disciplines will *get to them*. The interest in general systems theory, with its promise of umbrella-like relevance, is a sign of this growing awareness. What is probable, however, is that there will be very little progress towards comprehensive understanding (*i.e.*, multiple discipline synthesis) for many years. It is not likely that single disciplines coming together in suspicious alliance will generate the kind of synthesis required to make information comprehensible and useful. The alternative is a slow de novo development of a comprehensive behavioral science *discipline*. This is not the inter-disciplinary cooperative model that poses as a behavioral science but rather a new discipline, as was the case in the evolution of social psychology as distinct from either sociology or psychology.

The point of course is that such an evolution will be slow and far off. The corollary is that reasonably successful preventive programs, (of a primary sort), will also be far off. They may come after the development of a comprehensive language to describe the boundaries of discrete

behavior, and comprehensive theorems able to bring together validated causal variables from whatever parent
discipline. But until then, the primary preventer is in the
business of benevolent gambling.

Where does all of this bring us in our community orientation? Hopefully it will trim from our already overextended and illusory mandate, the expensive preoccupation
with primary prevention. Another way of saying this is
that preventive activities, should be of a limited sort when
performed by the community psychiatrist. And these
limited efforts should not include benevolent gambling.
When and if information (not speculation) is of a quality
and quantity to allow for *researchable* trial, then the community psychiatrist and others may provide the action arm
of such research. But the generation of the information is
most likely to come from scholars (with or without portfolio) who are able to take some distance from the service-
action identity of the community psychiatrist.

chapter 7

THE REQUIREMENTS:

The Five Roads to Heaven

Community Mental Health Center has thus far had to create its identity around five structural cornerstones placed within the geographic dimensions of the "catchment area." We have already considered some of the implications of the catchment area and shall now focus on those five structures: The out-patient services; in-patient services; day-hospital services; emergency services; consultation and education.

There is little question about the service orientation of the community mental health center when one realizes that four of the five mandated programs for a mental health center are direct care programs.[1] Some centers have nonetheless made social action their priority and have

1. Congress of the United States. Mental Retardation Facilities and Community Mental Health Centers Act of 1963. Public Law 88-164.

approached this either by distribution of staff and other resources to social action programming or by incorporating social action approaches within the service components themselves. There is considerable disagreement as to the most effective orientation for a community mental health center. Whether it will be a service to patients/clients or whether it will be primarily an instrument of social action is a question which we have considered in earlier sections, but one which will continue to be debated within the five structures and the catchment area regardless of other considerations. The chances of the community mental health center becoming a social action agency on a practical basis are much less than the chances of it becoming a service to patients operation. The odds are stacked in that direction because of the inherent functions of four of the five mandated components. In this section we will assume that the social action component of the center's operation resides elsewhere. Here we shall consider the five mandated services from a clinical perspective.

There is nothing inherently unique about these five components. Each has been a rather traditional piece of most psychiatric service facilities, particularly in training centers. The least familiar of them is the day hospital component. What is perhaps most unique about this five component package is the insistence that they be a package, *i.e.* a coordinated group of services geared towards care along the illness continuum from acute to chronic. The deficiency which the community mental health center was meant to correct was the uneven distribution of care facilities, affecting certain population groups particularly[2] and the uneven availability of more psychiatrically comprehensive service structures.[3] In the latter regard, it was apparent that outside of the private practice area, there was

2. Hollingshead, A. B., and Redlich, F. C.: *Social Class and Mental Illness,* New York: Wiley, 1958.
3. Joint Commission on Mental Illness and Health: *Action for Mental Health*, New York: Basic Books, 1961.

10

an over-emphasis on in-patient care without appropriate pre-hospital and post-hospital resources.[4] Emergency care was also significantly deficient. Day-care was seen as the logical compromise between in-patient and out-patient service.

It is important to realize the pedestrian quality of what was intended by mandating the essential five service components. There were gaps in the distribution of resources and gaps in the continuity of resources. The community mental health centers were clearly designed to fill those gaps. As pedestrian as that may seem, in the fragmented, virtuoso ethos of pre-existing psychiatric services, such a simple plan is nonetheless a dramatic departure.

The most legitimate problem in considering the five basic components has little to do with the social-action question. It is rather, how do these five components order themselves so as to provide comprehensive and continuous care? The approach to answering that question must start at a general level which supersedes the autonomy of any of the single components. This relates to our earlier consideration of the definitions of mental health and/or mental illness. The policy of the mental health center must first be settled as it relates to the service goals. Inherent in this process is the *exclusion* of various behavioral phenomena. We do *this* and *not that*. Or, we are concerned with *these* problems but not with *those* problems. From that point on, the five components must be addressed to those goals.

4. Prior to our institution of clinical services at the Temple University Community Mental Health Center (TCMHC), we undertook a survey of all psychiatric treatment facilities in the Philadelphia area. We looked at their records covering a one-year period and noted all patient contacts for persons residing within our catchment area. We saw a definite emphasis on hospital care, without complementary out-patient (*i.e.* pre-hospital or post-hospital) care. Berger, D. G. and Gardner, E. A.: *Use of Community Surveys in Mental Health Planning*. Presented at the American Public Health Association Meeting, November 1969. Submitted for publication.

Obviously, the fact that you have been mandated to start with those five components will influence your goal setting. This unfortunate putting of the cart before the horse has severely limited the goal setting process itself. But again, that objection will lead us far afield. If we assume that today's community psychiatrist has accepted the fact that he is *mandated* to provide five basic services and that he is mandated to care for the mentally ill (a concept which still allows for considerable interpretation), then certain issues follow logically.

CATEGORICAL VS. GENERAL APPROACH

In our earlier consideration of specialized and generalized resources a conclusion (of the author if not the reader) was that there is a place for approaching behavior from a categorical (or generic) perspective. In this approach we are concerned with problem categories, like alcoholism, mental retardation, psychosis, etc. An associated conclusion, however, was that there was also a place for approaching behavior from a general perspective. In this approach we are concerned with the more ubiquitous problems of a neurotic and psychosocial type. The categorical approach has the advantage of allowing one to more clearly demarcate the target problem groups and likewise to be more able to exclude other categorical problems *or* other general problems. If, for example, you indicate that the problems you will attempt to treat are the categories of psychosis, mental retardation and alcoholism, then your terrain is pretty well defined and many operational and policy decisions will flow logically. The other, more general approach, allows greater freedom but also provokes more ambiquity and difficulty in assignment of priority and resources.

The implicit expectation of most governmental funding bodies is that the community mental health centers will at *least* provide services for those categorical problems which have traditionally been the responsibility of public concern (government), meaning psychosis and mental retardation at the minimum. This implicit, and in some instances explicit, mandating of a categorical approach for mental health centers, carries with it an enormous consequence that has not yet dawned on many newer community mental health programs. It is simply this: doing a good job of comprehensive and continuous care of the psychotics and mental retardates of a base population group of from 75,000 to 200,000, may very likely absorb every available manhour of resource . . . and then some. There is even some question as to how well both categories can be served by one center.

To add other categories onto the service goals and/or to become an open-ended general service is virtually to guarantee a reduction of quality across the board . . . simply on the basis of deficient resources.[5] All this leads to an important starting point: service goals of a community mental health center (if governmentally funded) must begin with those categories which fall under public responsibility (*e.g.* psychosis and mental retardation). Expansion of goals beyond those basic categories should be considered only after the pattern of service use and its adequacy for the basic categories have been tested in practice. Furthermore, expansion of service goals beyond the basic categories should be from a categorical perspective.

The use of the categorical approach in adding service goals has several rationales. In the first place we have had to begin with a categorical approach by implicit and often explicit mandate. That carries with it an enormous service commitment. From that point on it is imperative that further service commitments are manageable so as to avoid

5. The acceptance of the fact that quality of care would probably suffer in the catchment area—community mental health center romance, was noted by Zusman in his discussion of the catchment area concept: Zusman, J.: Design of Catchment Areas for Community Mental Health Services, *Archives of General Psychiatry*, 5: 568—573, 1969.

overcommitment. The most practical way to do that is to work with explicit categories and to avoid the open-door implications of a general approach.

Another reason for this approach has to do with my oft repeated plea for task clarity. As a service program grows by categorical increments the tasks for therapists become more clearly defined and their specialization strengths can be best utilized. Eventually, assuming a continuing growth, the total service program will have approached a general intake character by including more and more types of problems.

The hooker in all of this is a persistently nagging possibility that very few community mental health centers will enjoy enough longevity to see them far beyond services to the basic categories. It seems axiomatic for governmentally-funded health programs never to get beyond the squeakiest wheel.

The service components will now be considered from the rather narrow perspective that has been painfully elaborated to this point.

EMERGENCY SERVICES

Emergency psychiatric service is one of the most necessary of the five components, the most difficult program to mount, the most taxing program to maintain, the most expensive to run, and is the most likely to explode in your face.[6] The interesting phenomenon thus far in the development of emergency services within community mental health centers is that they are developing in the least productive way. They are small, understaffed, overworked and

6. My first task upon entering the community mental health field four years ago was to establish a psychiatric emergency unit. That unit, called the Crisis Center, has borne the brunt of the difficult clinical load of the Mental Health Center. It has suffered enormously, in its personnel stresses, morale fluctuations, space shortages, and expansive expectations. It proved to be the most needed of services (contacts numbered 20 per day) and one of the most vulnerable to criticism.

in constant danger of extinction. This is probably more apparent in large urban mental health centers because lower class persons are more prone to use emergency facilities. But if suburban mental health centers had publicized and adequately staffed emergency units, Parkinson's Law would see to their rapid over-utilization as well.

The first orienting statement about the emergency service is that it should be the nerve center of the mental health center. It should be the common portal of entry for all patients to the care system and it should be prepared to function diagnostically and therapeutically within a strict time span. It should work in concert with a patient advocacy system housed within the emergency area and therefore be intimately related to reporting and recording systems. It should be staffed by the most experienced and sophisticated of staff and have a dispositional authority invested in it. It should have pleasant and efficient space with a holding bed capacity dependent on (a) daily utilization rate for the emergency service and (b) availability of in-patient beds for the categories serviced in the emergency service.[7] It should be as close as possible to a full range medical emergency department of a general hospital (contiguous if possible).[8] Let us expand on some of these points.

7. The Crisis Center began with 3 beds which were quickly inundated. Over a four-year period the bed-capacity was increased to 6, with considerable pressure from staff to expand to as many as 12 beds. It seemed clear that we could have expanded to 20 beds and still have experienced pressure for more. The vital link in determining emergency bed need is the availability of immediate in-patient beds.

8. The Crisis Center was housed on the first floor of a three floor row house, approximately three blocks from the main emergency department of Temple University Hospital. This caused a constant gap in communication effectiveness between the two departments and severely limited the quality and quantity of general medical expertise available for Crisis Center patients.

Since a community mental health center attempts to be more than a cumulative collection of individual therapists, and assumes a comprehensive system approach, it must follow the dynamics of systems. One of the characteristics of systems is their centralized control. The parts of the system may be far flung, but if those parts are to work together according to some overriding plan, then there must be a centralizing of control of those parts. In a patient care system where a series of far flung system parts are expected to work together and where a patient might be expected to proceed from one part to another, the need for centralized control is no less urgent. We have already indicated the need for a patient advocacy system and its potential role as mediator and programmer between the patient and the system. It follows that the patient advocacy system be involved from the beginning and so it is reasonable that the patient advocacy system be at a logical entry portal to the full range of services. There is only one portal of entry that can be consistently used as an exclusive portal of entry and that is the emergency service. If someone is entering the system for the first time under urgent circumstances, he most likely will enter through the emergency service. If someone is entering the system under less urgent circumstances, he can do so through the intake of the emergency-patient advocacy service. This allows for initial diagnostic and therapeutic planning and disposition to the appropriate specialized service component.

Under this arrangement we have a sophisticated team responsible for problem analysis and therapeutic planning and disposition at the intake portal whether intake is of an emergency type or not. Whereas it is possible to have separate emergency service and central intake, it is not as efficient. Other possibilities include multiple intake portals (also separated from the emergency service) as might be the case in a center which utilized satellite locations. This arrangement suffers because of the difficulty in reproducing sophisticated functions (emergency as well as diagnostic) and making them available to multiple locations.[9] All things considered, it seems preferable to combine emergency and intake (of the patient advocacy sort) in a centralized location and with collaborative function.

A planning, coordinating and dispositional operation requires that authority be vested in it. It means that the other service units to whom patients will be sent must understand the hierarchy of decision making as it relates to patient disposition and therapeutic plan. When the various service components are allowed to function with a high degree of autonomy, particularly in reference to whom they will treat and whom they will not, then you are dealing with an uneasy confederation and not a system.[10]

There is a danger as well as an advantage in having holding beds in an emergency service. It is helpful to be able to delay disposition until adequate information has been obtained and holding beds allow for that delay. It is also helpful to be able to initiate intense therapy in certain cases with the avoidance of hospitalization a greater possibility. But it is also possible to become a repository for the impossible dispositions. There are many problem categories that simply do not have adequate resources for their

9. The clinical services of TCMHC experimented with a single entry system as well as a multiple entry system. The latter system was an inevitable consequence of a clinical decentralization program started in the third year which began to emphasize satellite clinical settings. It made standardization of quality and overall approach very difficult to maintain. Although it made access to the Center more convenient for the patient, it made his over-all long range care less than adequate.

10. Temple Community Mental Health Center began its development with strong leadership within each component unit of the Center. Each developed with its own élan, its own orientation and its own sense of hierarchy. This innate competition allowed for strong units but also generated their uneasy alliance in pursuit of common goals. Because of persisting ambiguity regarding these goals, the fragmentation of the component units was reinforced to the detriment of the overall clinical program.

care. The senile patient is a glaring example. Avoiding the argument of whether senility is a psychiatric problem or not, it is a fact that senile patients, without adequate living arrangements, frequently end up in emergency services. This trend seems directly proportional to the level of poverty of the patient. The same general rule seems to apply to various stages of mental retardation, debilitated alcoholics, and psychotic children and young adolescents.[11]

The threat of repository is a predictable price to pay for developing a reputation for unqualified open-endedness. The problem of where to draw the line is different for the emergency service than it is for the remaining service components. The emergency service need not assume a continuing responsibility for patient care, with the exception of its patient advocacy arm, and the latter is more properly a monitoring function rather than patient care function. Because of this ability to avoid cumulative treatment loads it is feasible for an emergency service to be more comprehensive and hence more open-ended than the mental health center at large. Whether it can afford to be truly open-ended, *i.e.* with no exclusions for service, depends almost entirely on its space and personnel resources. It also depends on the availability, in the community at large, of resources for those problems which will not be dealt with in other service components of the mental health center.

Regardless of the direction the emergency service takes within a mental health center, it almost invariably becomes a maintenance problem. The problems generated around emergency services seem to be directly related to the degree of frustration faced by the staff of the emergency service in carrying out their daily tasks. When a service component finds itself unable to cope adequately with the demands placed on it, there ensues a gradual (and at times

11. One of the quickest ways to learn about a community's resources is to establish an open door emergency unit (as was the case with the Crisis Center) and struggle with the dispositional nightmares that inevitably develop.

explosive) unraveling of personnel responsibility, initiative and tolerance. No service component is more vulnerable to this drowning phenomenon than the emergency service.[12] Faced with an around-the-clock mandate and with a relatively unpredictable work load, it must have a staffing pattern that allows all personnel some respite from the stress. It must also have clarity regarding its mandate. Who qualifies as a patient and who does *not* must be reasonably clear. Dispositional alternatives must be available for all the categorical problems it is likely to face.

In many community mental health programs, emergency services are conceptualized in very modest terms. Often a single physician is "on-call" (a euphemism for being reluctantly available) and he sees his role as being limited to rapid diagnosis and *rapid* disposition. Treatment is considered the responsibility of the referred-to resource. Very little effort goes into intensive initial exploration of the problem. The emphasis is on rapid turnover and on triage. Such "quick and dirty" procedures are logical consequences of an unwillingness to invest in emergency services. And much of the unwillingness to invest in emergency services is prompted by a predictable unwillingness of many professionals to work in so stressful a situation. It is an unfortunate legacy of prior emergency room experience that such work seems invariably frustrating and overwhelming. Most emergency services become compromises between what they should be like and what they shouldn't be like and the net result tends more towards the latter rather than the former. And so we see a continuing cycle of stressful experience and an eventual reluctance to be exposed to such stress in the future.

12. The relationship between the staff of the Crisis Center (on the firing line) and the administrative-policy leadership (in distant offices) was frequently strained by the feelings of the former that they were being forced to provide "inhumane care" and not adequately staffed nor equipped. The limitations of space confounded the issues. In general the position of the firing line staff was more realistic than was that of the policy setting group, of which I was a participant.

There is a further factor of stress on personnel that has little to do with the quantity of the work load. It has to do with poor training in the area of the psychiatric emergency. Residents in many training programs have little if any experience in the techniques and rationales of crisis or emergency care. Many residency programs bend over backward to avoid such experiences and when it is impossible to avoid entirely, the resident is assigned with apology and often "compensation" for this unfortunate necessity.[13] The inadequacy of professional training plus the insufficiency of professional manpower compounds the problem of proper staffing of an emergency service.

The tendency seems to be contrary to what I feel is the optimum pattern for emergency service. Rather than small, apologetic and anemic, emergency services should be comprehensive, sophisticated, and central to the entire service program of a community mental health center. It has long been known that the fall out rates or the "do-not-show" rates for psychiatric out-patients are quite high after an initial enthusiasm. This enthusiasm seems to last for three or four visits. It seems quite appropriate then, to assign a priority in personnel distribution and secondary supports to those component services that are concerned with the early phases of a patient's experience in a psychiatric care program.

IN-PATIENT SERVICES

Because community psychiatry has made much of its comprehensive approach and its systematic concern for continuity, it has generated an anti-hospitalization philos-

13. I quickly became one of the most unpopular men on campus with the opening of the Crisis Center. I had expected that residents would come to see their work in an emergency unit as professionally profitable and exciting. Whereas this view proved to be generally true, it became so only after they received compensation beyond their usual residency stipend. In the interim, the department of psychiatry was faced with a very militant and angry reluctance by the residents to be thrown into Daniel's cave (Panzetta's folly).

ophy. Some feel that success can be measured by declining hospitalization rates or by shorter stays in the hospital. The shameful tradition of many mental hospitals, particularly of large public institutions, still reminds us of the dreadful plight of patients in the days before and after Pinel. Hospitals have long seemed custodial warehouses for societal rejects, ... akin to land-locked ships of fools. Despite remarkable improvement in the quality of care for in-patients, particularly since the development of psychiatric wards within general hospitals, the in-patient phase of care is still anathema and rapid discharge is a persistent goal. This is certainly understandable, particularly when the in-patient facility lacks program, personnel and hospitable surroundings. But the push towards "return to the community" is no less urgent when the in-patient facility is model.

The primary argument seems to be that a hospital setting is basically unnatural and a patient must learn proper adaptation within the natural setting of his home or community environment. It is hard to argue against the danger of regressive dependency by patients who are given a prolonged sanctuary in a hospital setting. Anyone with experience in such settings can quickly recognize the reality of that danger. But on the other hand, experience also convincingly tells us that, for many patients, a temporary sanctuary from the stresses of life can be enough to restore affective and cognitive balance. It can be a very valuable and necessary experience.[14]

If the latter is true, then it is naive to hold either a high

14. Temple Community Mental Health Center had recourse to three separate and widely divergent in-patient resources. There was the in-patient floor of the University hospital, where at any one time, up to a third of patients were from the catchment area. There was the Temple unit at Eastern Pennsylvania Psychiatric Institute, where the emphasis was on teaching and research. There was the Temple unit at Philadelphia State Hospital, staffed by Temple Community Mental Health Center personnel. The State Hospital unit was the mainstay of our in-patient resource and was our tangible manifestation of interest in the welfare of our patients throughout the illness continuum from acute to chronic.

or low hospitalization rate as evidence of good or bad service. In and of itself a hospitalization rate is meaningless. Certainly it can be manipulated to one's wishes by either pushing the discharge rate or by making admission more difficult. These are more realistically administrative devices to achieve *administrative goals* and not to be confused with therapeutic devices to achieve clinical goals.

The more relevent issue is how good are the in-patient program and its personnel and towards what goals do they strive? If the answer to the latter part of that question is "the rapid return of patients to the community," then the entire in-patient operation is a revolving door dedicated to fewer staff headaches. It is unlikely that an in-patient program would in fact be entirely motivated by a rapid disposition philosophy. It could, if forced, no doubt articulate many concrete clinical goals which order the component's operation. These goals, however, are often obscured by the premium placed on rapid turnover and the illusory benefits of "return to the community."

The development of clinical goals for the in-patient component of a community mental health center cannot be achieved in isolation. These goals must reflect the overall clinical goals of the center and must be carefully related to the cooperative roles of the emergency service and outpatient service. What *part* of the *whole* will become the responsibility of the in-patient component? That is the quality of the relevant question. With this broader perspective, "return to the community" is replaced by considerations of pre-hospital resources and post-hospital resources.[15]

15. The clinical goals of the Temple unit at Philadelphia State Hospital, were modest and realistic. The orientation was to reduce or remove socially dysfunctional symptoms (primarily psychotic) so as to permit a return to the community. The expectation of the staff was that ongoing support and further symptom oriented treatment would be provided by the out-patient service of Temple Community Mental Health Center. The State Hospital Unit was some 25 miles distant from Temple Community Mental Health Center. The discontinuity between the in-patient
(Continued on next page.)

There is a further issue, particularly relevant to community psychiatry, that has to do with its comprehensive mandate. The expectation is that in-patient service will extend from acute care through chronic and even custodial care. The pattern seems to be the following: The community mental health centers are placing a priority on acute in-patient service with chronic and custodial care either being ignored or left to existing institutions which are already doing a poor job. It may be necessary to do precisely that for survival sake alone, since the resources for doing everything are as plentiful as mesozoic era dinosaurs. It is quite reasonable to distribute limited resources to those types of in-patient services that are most likely to be effective and which fit into the overall clinical program of the center.

Despite the best laid plans, however, it is inevitable that chronic and custodial care facilities are and will be required to complement any legitimate comprehensive mental health program. Where they will come from and what they will do may be unfolded in the near future . . . . . if the whole community mental health movement can be sustained long enough.

OUT-PATIENT SERVICES

The bulk of the ongoing responsibility for patient care within a community mental health center falls to the out-patient component. It is potentially less confined by the structural requirements of emergency and in-patient services and can be experimental in a great number of ways. As with the other components, however, it will not be an efficient and complementary service unless its own goals

unit and out-patient unit suggested that more than distance separated them.

Out-patient staff tended to see the patient as having been rushed out of the hospital without adequate treatment or preparation. The in-patient staff tended to see the out-patient staff as disorganized and unwilling or unable to follow-up on patient needs. Both units lived within their own parochial borders and demonstrated (as if it were needed) the need for supervening centralized programming and control.

and methods are fitted into the overall clinical goals of the center.[16]

There are two major questions regarding out-patient services that we shall consider here: what should the service do? where should it be done? The first question could conceivably be overwhelming if we allow ourselves to be seduced into a consideration of the pros and cons of one therapeutic school against some other. It should be sufficiently clear at this time that there has occurred a proliferation of various therapeutic techniques with considerable confusion as to which technique claims superiority for which problem. As occurs too often, emphasis is placed on the technique without sufficient clarity as to the problem *for which* it is effective. The point to be made here is that, *rather* than start with this technique or that, we should start with this problem or that problem. We should begin, as has been suggested earlier, with a designation of which problems shall be included in our therapeutic goals. In the community mental health center these may very well be mandated for us (*e.g.* schizophrenia and mental retardation) in which case we start with those problems and then work towards the techniques we choose to apply to those problems. If for no other reason, the clarity of problems approach will at least help in whatever therapy evaluation studies the center is able to carry out.

By and large most community mental health centers have had to spread the responsibility for therapy beyond the psychiatrist to other professionals and paraprofessionals.[17] One result has been to undermine a standardized expectation of therapy. Each therapist goes at it with his own idiosyncratic talent, training, philosophy and technique. This phenomenon is not too unusual nor is it

16. I was responsible for the development of out-patient services (Psycho-social Clinic) and because of the numerous modifications in design and operation of that service, it is historically summarized in the appendix of this book.

17. Levenson, A. I.: Staffing, in Grunebaum, H. (Edit.): *The Practice of Community Mental Health*, Boston: Little, Brown and Co., 1970.

peculiar to community mental health centers because most psychiatric clinics, public as well as private, university as well as not, have been characterized by a poorly standardized therapeutic delivery system.

This may be overly ambitious or too premature, but nonetheless it seems reasonable to plead for some degree of therapeutic standardization as well as problem standardization. How this will be worked out will depend on the clarity and reasonableness of leadership, for it is predictable that therapists (regardless of professional or nonprofessional status) will balk at being urged to use standardized therapy.

But presuming we could cope with the resistance and were in a position to use standardized therapy for standardized problems, how should we proceed? Perhaps we should back up first before considering that question. Standardized therapy makes no sense unless there is a standardized way of considering problems. This means a revision of nomenclature. A psychosocial nomenclature must be developed which avoids the pitfalls of trying to organize itself around etiology. An etiologically grounded nomenclature is at best a very distant goal. We are in no way near such a development. The nomenclature might be organized around one of several hypothetic concepts which would have direct interventional relevance. The decision as to the direction to take in developing a nomenclature is really dependent on one's philosophic orientation as to how and why humans behave as they do.[18] The discontinuity between our standard nomenclature and the

18. A nomenclature, to be productive, must have internal logical consistency. The DSMII nomenclature is a good example of logical inconsistency. It has no unifying frame of reference. There are numerous possibilities in the development of a nomenclature because it simply indicates "a way of looking at" rather than "the only way of looking at." It therefore suggests using basic *assumptions* and identifying them as assumptions. The use and identification of assumptions can be considered philosophic. Philosophy, not in dogmatic trappings, but in legitimate exploration, is all scientists ultimately do in their initial hypothesizing.

various treatment approaches is due to the heterogenous input used to develop the nomenclature vs. the homogenous orientation of each group of therapists. The nomenclature is a committee compromise and as such provides little coherence for a treatment delivery system. It is a burden, but nonetheless a necessity, that the delivery system advocates spend initial time and effort in developing their own nomenclature. If they are of the learning theory orientation, then their nomenclature should organize itself around the therapeutic differences for each behavioral item in the nomenclature. The same applies for other viewpoints, therapeutic systems, schools or whatever. If persons in community psychiatry find themselves with a rather disjointed and crazy-quilt sense of nomenclature to start with and *cannot* or *will not* work to reorder that nomenclature so that it will be more systematic and have interventional relevance, then they will have failed in a primary task. They will have failed to put clinical problems into a systematic conceptual scheme so that a systematic delivery system can be constructed. Such behavior is like constructing an electron microscope to study the stars.

We may have backed ourselves into a corner. We have developed an orientation that places high priority on the development of a coordinated systematic delivery system with emphasis on task clarity. That has led us to recognize the need for an organization of problems into a nomenclature which is systematic and logically consistent and which complements the delivery system. Most community psychiatry advocates have been involved, up to their earlobes, in the work of the delivery system in its gross dimensions. Some have gone further and have been able to clarify the discrete tasks to a limited extent. But the latter process cannot proceed to an efficient level unless the nomenclature issue is resolved. Very few have been willing or able to devote their energies in this direction. The delivery systems are coming before the nomenclature systems: the cart is well ahead of the horse.

This issue has particular relevance in our consideration of out-patient services because it is here that the tone of the entire community mental health center is set. If the center is truly operating as a system, rather than a discrete group of autonomous units, then the out-patient service sets the pace. It has less structural predeterminism than the other service components and so is freer to develop the clinical orientation of the center.

This brings us to a peculiar answer to the first question: what should the service do? It should do what *it has decided to do*, based on its development of a *standardized nomenclature*. If it has not developed such a nomenclature then it should cease the masquerade as a service component of a broader service delivery system. If a center has decided on limited clinical problems, (for argument's sake let us again say schizophrenia and mental retardation), then it still has the task of developing a nomenclature which organizes these two very broad clinical syndromes into more discrete sub units of behavior with each unit having certain interventional implications. That is a hard task *but* if it cannot be done then it is foolish to think it possible to develop a treatment system which includes multiple therapists, techniques and facilities.

The second question (where should the work of the out-patient service be done?) has a geographic flavor. It has become a relevant question in community psychiatry because of the geographic orientation of the whole movement. A logical extension of the concept of catchment area is the concept of sub-catchment area. Given an area with population of 75,000 to 200,000 the stage is set for subdividing that population into "more workable" groupings. The problem of course is that no one knows how big a "workable" group is. Some of the neighborhood health centers (of OEO sponsorship) work with two census tracts and with variable populations of 25,000 to 50,000 persons. The satellite activities of mental health centers vary radically and there seems to be no consensus as to what an ideal size is for what function.

A more reasonable approach to justify the decentralization of services is based on convenience for patients. The closer a service is to one's residence, so the argument goes, the more readily it will be used. It is also argued that moving "out into the community" proves the good will of the service and enables the service and "community people" to develop mutually helpful relationships.

The validity of the above assertions can certainly be challenged but their refutation as well as their proof is not ultimately determined by facts. Arguments for or against are educated guesses at best for the issue of centralization vs. decentralization is as old as ancient Rome and even older. The centralization vs. decentralization controversy seems to be invariably argued on the two issues of reasonable distance for consumer and administrative manageability. Both of these issues are quite relative and do not lend themselves to absolute guidelines. It seems reasonably clear, that as one seeks an ideal unit of population (neighborhood, town, city, metropolitan area, region) he finds that there is no one ideal. The ideal unit varies according to why one seeks an ideal unit.[19] For the public school system an ideal unit may be regional so as to incorporate the resources of city and suburban areas. A grocer may wish to focus on a neighborhood unit, while a supermarket chain may see a city as the ideal unit. And so it goes. For a community mental health center the decision as to the ideal unit of population, should *follow*, not precede, the decision as to the functions of the individual center. In the community mental health movement how-

19. This has been true in the new interest being accorded the family as a therapeutic unit. Neither the family nor any other unit (person, couple, psyche, brain, etc.) is "better" than any other. The unit one *chooses* to focus on is relative to the rationale behind the choice.

ever, the fundamental population unit has been mandated at the start. This certainly influences the setting of goals (as has been noted elsewhere). If the goals are variations around the basic themes of comprehensive and continuous care for selected problem categories, then it is harder to see why satellite operations (*i.e.* further decentralization) are justified, except for the strictly geographic convenience of the patient. The administrative duplication that goes into satellite programming and the dilution of available staff can easily compromise the strength of the basic clinical program.

If a centralized clinical program suffers because transportation lines to the center are inadequate or inconvenient, then satellite programming becomes more desirable but it may very well be at the expense of the overall program. Both quality control and quantity control become much more difficult with a decentralized operation.

There is another valid rationale for the development of satellite operations. Certain catchment areas may have within their boundaries rather discrete groups with homogenous class or ethnic characteristics. When this occurs it is safe to say that their buying patterns (consumer life styles) may vary from the catchment area at large. Variations in the clinical service style may be called for to maintain consumer attraction and this may be more easily accomplished using a discrete satellite unit within this group's area.

Much could be said regarding the advisability of clinical services within the home setting, *i.e.* home visiting, but we shall restrict our comments to only a few points. Except in rather specific instances, the plan to provide home care as an ongoing strategy, is not wise. It is inefficient in the distribution of staff time and more intrusive to family equilibrium than we choose to admit. There is great advantage to home visiting as an early diagnostic procedure because the quality and quantity of helpful data for diagnostic formulation is frequently enhanced. There is also promise in home visiting as practiced so successfully by visiting nurses. But here the focus would be on maintenance contacts, usually to monitor gross symptoms and signs and to insure control of a maintenance drug program.

The compromise between the "convenience" of home visiting (for the patient) and the "inconvenience" (for the staff) must be struck in a way which serves the clinical goals of the program. Any prior statement that says it is good to do a great deal of home visiting must be challenged. "Home visiting for what purpose?" Do those purposes serve the ultimate clinical goals of the center? Some studies have asserted that home visiting is a feasible way to reduce hospitalization, particularly for chronic conditions such as schizophrenia or in chronic brain syndrome.[20] The use of a home visiting program for a specific purpose (such as maintenance of schizophrenics) makes good sense. The objection raised here regarding home visiting refers only to the practice of attaching a positive value to home visiting for its own sake. It is the indiscriminate glorification of the home visit that must be avoided.

PARTIAL HOSPITALIZATION SERVICES

The partial hospitalization program is the least familiar of the mandated services. We have generally used an all or none approach to hospitalization without the compromise which is afforded by a day-hospital or night-hospital. The innovative aspect of this partial hospital service is its provision of structured program for periods of time which are in excess of the usual out-patient programs and less than the usual in-patient programs. It is certainly much closer to in-patient care, in that a patient is likely to spend greater blocks of time in a structured in-house program. It tends

20. Pasamanick, B. Scarpitti, F. R. and Dinitz, S.: *Schizophrenics in the Community*, New York: Appleton-Century-Crofts, 1967.

to provide sanctuary certainly to a much greater extent than does the relatively infrequent out-patient contact.

Its advantages are thought to come from its flexibility and its greater impact on behavior. It is flexible in that patients can continue some degree of "normal" transaction with their environment. It has greater impact in that patients are exposed for extended periods to the therapeutic program. In the latter instance, however, it should be pointed out that there is no assurance that behavioral modification has any connection to the duration of therapeutic effort.

The program structure itself can vary widely and existing day-hospital or night-hospital (or week-end hospital) programs are quite diverse in their goals and methods of operation.[21/22/23] As a general statement, however, it can be asserted that the partial hospitalization program should be an integrated part of the total clinical service program, extending from emergency care through out-patient and in-patient care. How partial hospital services will *complement* the total clinical service package is the relevant question, with the understanding that there are multiple possible roles, providing the one selected does in fact complement the total clinical program.

21. Temple Community Mental Health Center has operated a partial hospital program which has included day-hospital services, (called "Our Place"), night-hospital services and week-end hospital services. An excellent review of partial hospital practices and a conceptual and operational analysis of "Our Place" can be found in Glaser, F. B.: *Our Place: Design for a Day Program,* American Journal of Orthopsychiatry, 5, 827−841, 1969.
22. Glasscote, R. M., Kraft, A. M., Glassman, S. M. and Jepson, W. W.: *Partial Hospitalization for the Mentally Ill*, Washington, D.C.: The Joint Information Service of the American Psychiatric Association and the National Association for Mental Health, 1969.
23. Chen, R., Healey, J. and Williams, H. V.: *Partial Hospitalization-Problems, Purposes, and Changing Objectives*, Topeka: Robert Sanders, 1969.

CONSULTATION AND EDUCATION

There is a great deal written about the content and the process of consultation.[24][25][26][27] We shall not go over that ground again here. The entire area of psychiatric consultation and education is hardly new. What is new is the attempt to intensify the quantity of this activity by making it an essential part of each community mental health center. Of the five mandated components, C & E is the most unstructured and potentially innovative. It can move in a variety of directions and the C & E programs of community mental health centers are as varied as the number of centers.

In general C & E goals can be ordered around one or more of the three levels of preventive programming. Some seem interested in consulting to agencies of secondary prevention,[28] some to agencies of tertiary prevention.[29] Still others attempt to consult to agencies or institutions which they feel are instrumental in primary prevention.[30] The most traditional consultation is probably aimed at the secondary prevention level. Presumably there is an expertise which is communicable and caretakers of the emotionally disturbed can benefit from such expertise. Each consultant brings his own idiosyncratic set of experiences, training, bias and talent into the consultation process and

24. Caplan, G.: *Concepts of Mental Health and Consultation*, Washington: U.S. Children's Bureau, Publication No. 373, U.S. Government Printing Office, 1959.
25. Caplan, G.: *Principles of Preventive Psychiatry*, New York: Basic Books, 1964.
26. Caplan, G.: Types of Mental Health Consultation, *American Journal of Orthopsychiatry*, 33:470–481, 1963.
27. Mendel, W. M. and Solomon, P., (eds.): *The Psychiatric Consultation*, New York: Grune & Stratton, 1968.
28. Caplan, G.: op. cit., 1963.
29. Hader, M.: The Psychiatrist As a Consultant to the Social Worker in a Home For the Aged, *Journal of the American Geriatric Society*, 14, 407–413, 1966.
30. Caplan, G.: op. cit., 1964.

dispenses liberal quantities to the less expert. A social worker presumably has been trained to an extent which allows for helpful interaction with troubled persons. But there are boundaries to the social worker's competence in therapy (or so it has been legislated) and so when at the boundary lines, help must be secured. Psychiatrists, however, are expert at responding to calls for help whether by social workers, nurses, politicians, educators, city planners or patients. Their stock in trade is a verbal conglomerate glued with tight theory and implacable faith. There is literally no problem that cannot be "explained" or "understood" from a psychodynamic point of view. Armed with new "understanding" the social worker, or whoever is the fortunate recipient of the consultation, can carry on with greater tolerance and sophistication. It would be interesting to know what the net effect on the care to the client is from the consultant's expertise. The consultation process no doubt has an influence on the caretaker (consultee) and in many instances it no doubt works to the ultimate advantage of the client (or patient). What may in fact be most crucial in the entire interaction is not the communication of information from consultant to consultee, but rather the ubiquitous therapeutic (to the consultee) process between consultant and consultee. Reassurance and reinforcement of innate consultee talents may be the real stuff of successful consultation.

But if that is so, then certain things follow regarding the ultimate efficiency of the consulting community psychiatrist. He is spreading the wealth and so should be concerned about who is receiving the wealth. If his consultation enables others to provide clinical service in a more satisfactory way, then he is a resource and, in this world of short supply, the utilization of resource becomes very important. We are again leading to a rather predictable starting point. Since a community mental health center starts with explicit goals (or at least should), then the consultant's role must be part of that goal-oriented program.

The direct clinical services, aiming at specific clinical goals *need the help* of a consultation vanguard concerned with those *same* clinical goals. The common experience shows a discontinuity between the clinical services and the C & E component. While the clinical services may be in hot pursuit of (let us say) schizophrenia, the consultants may be out consulting to neurotic problems. In the unlikely event it has escaped the reader's attention up to now, it should be made clear that I favor bullets rather than buckshot. The name of the game is comprehensive and continuous but that does not equal diffuse and eternal. If the mental health center has target problems, then the entire program, including C & E, should be addressed to those target problems.

This leads us to activities of C & E which not only miss the targets of secondary and tertiary prevention established for the center, but avoid them entirely, in pursuit of a nobler goal, primary prevention. We have touched on this at several points in the preceding text and in most instances I have held my head in pain. To be sure, efforts in consultation and education work have great promise. They are addressed to broad social institutions and complicated social dilemmas. Both social institutions and dilemmas have multiple determining factors, not the least of which is psychologic. It seems to follow then that psychologic sophistication, as carried in the consultant's portfolio, should be communicated to the would-be makers and shapers of social institutions and would-be curers of social problems. These makers, shapers, and curers are the schools, police, courts, political structures, urban planners, and wherever power congregates to shape the lives of masses. This is primary prevention aimed at the institutional level.

The problem with institutional consultation as practiced by the community psychiatrist, is that, too often, he is ignorant about the institution to which he consults (or hopes to consult). He enters the consultative role with a benevolent arrogance which expects that institutional rigidity and policy will melt in his presence. His words are pearls thrown before swine.

The influencing of social institutions does not come from outside expertise, short of revolutionary militance. It comes from internal policy and internal dynamics of the institutions. To presume that one can influence a police department by providing an educational program for recruits is to badly underestimate the system of reinforcement of status quo which operates within that organization, and in fact within most organizations. Systems are changed from within or destroyed from without.

This merely suggests that consultation programs aimed at broad institutions are extraordinarily difficult at best. They require, at the outset, a great deal of information (public and private) about the target institution and they require an entrée into the very blood and guts of that institution's life. If those conditions can be met then perhaps it is worthwhile to pursue the goal of institutional modification.

Another variation of primary preventive consultation, or more correctly education, is addressed to non-institutional social targets. Influencing the voting process, acting for remedial housing policy, advocating action on the issues of poverty, crime and racism are examples of this type of preventive work.[31] These efforts are invariably tied to a political and social philosophy which orders them and provides them with elan. The degree of militancy or agitation

31. The C & E component of Temple Community Mental Health Center was never adequately related to the clinical goals of the center. They saw their role as broader in scope and fell under the spell of prevention of social inequity. With this orientation, they became significantly involved in such work as rent strikes with escrow accounts, stimulation of voter registration, and other political activism. They also were instrumental in more clinically related programs such as police training, educational experiences for clergy in mental health, and training of indigenous personnel.

attached to such programming varies enormously and is related primarily to the idiosyncratic personality and charisma of its leadership.

Here we are in a no man's land because the ideology drowns the rational methodology. It is possible for any man to sit in sublime isolation atop a green mountain and articulate a social philosophy. This social philosophy then takes on goods and evils. It is logical to then isolate the evil and plot its eradication from the fabric of social life. If a thousand men sat on a thousand green mountains and concocted a thousand social philosophies, it would probably be astounding to see the similarities in their ideological evils. If the thousand men, with their thousand philosophies shared their thoughts, they might very likely agree on the top twenty social evils. When they discussed how to eradicate those evils, they would probably revert to one thousand separate, and in some instances mutually exclusive, solutions. Men agree on ideology much more readily than they do on methodology. And this is the paradox which sets good men against each other. Eventually their antagonism clouds the fact that they may share the same ideology, may want the same good or the eradication of the same evil. They accuse each other and compete, either combatively or within social rules.

This fact of methodologic individualism provides great tension within any program which sets out to influence non-institutional social targets. If there are such goals within a community mental health center, prepare for a stormy trip. The storm may get severe enough to upset the entire program, including the clinical parts. To avoid such internal splintering, an unsavory condition must exist. Unhappily the leadership must be unchallenged and it must be charismatic and prophetic. If the mental health center can achieve that kind of religious coherence, then it may be able to pursue social targets with unity of purpose and method. But it will be just another grandiose illusion in the last analysis.

chapter 8

A THEORETICAL PERSPECTIVE:
Causal and Action Models*

A growing appreciation for the limitations of psychoanalytic theory has developed within recent years. Although still the most comprehensive and fecund theory of
human psychology, it has left important gaps in both
theory and practice which have pushed us on in new directions, ever in search of more inclusive models. It has been
accepted as a fundamental principle of scientific theory
construction that "if you don't know why certain things
happen then invent a mechanism (in accordance with the
view you take of how the world works)—but it is better
still if you find out how nature really works."[1] This, of

*This chapter is based on a previously published paper with some
modification.

Causal and Action Models in Social Psychiatry, in *Archives of
General Psychiatry*, March 1967.

1. Harré, R.: *Theories and Things*, New York: Sheed & Ward Ltd.,
   1961.

course, is the process of model construction. In science we strive for the development of laws governing the phenomena to be "explained." In the realm of behavior and its psychological roots we are deeply committed to the construction of models since we are a long distance from the realization of laws. What we know of the mechanisms of behavior (*i.e.*, not on the level of model, but on the level of true nature) is a function of our limited instruments; the rest is filled with models.

The emerging facts and models can be ordered around different frames of reference, from the neuroanatomic through the neurophysiologic, the psychologic, the psychosocial, the social, the sociocultural, the cultural, etc. As in the conceptualizations of von Bertalanffy, we can refer to these as "systems."[2] One measure of the degree of worth of any model in any system relates to its usefulness in providing a basis for understanding and for action either within the same system as the model or within another system. The degree to which a model enables predictable success in multiple systems determines to a significant degree its theoretical and pragmatic value. So then, the psychoanalytic model of mental apparatus (*i.e.* id, ego, superego) allows us a reasonable degree of predictability regarding the behavior of man as long as we remain focused at the proper system of abstraction, in the psychologic system. As we move toward the somatic, id or ego psychology is less relevant because it tells us little about the reticular activating system or the neurophysiology of dreaming. But then again, Hebb's neurologic model[3] does not help predict on a level where forces for subcultural conformity clash with forces for status enhancement. And further, Parson's theory of socialization[4] does not help speculations regarding delusional thought.

2. von Bertalanffy, L.: *Problems of Life: An Evaluation of Modern Biological Thought*, New York: John Wiley & Sons, Inc., 1952.
3. Hebb, D. O.: *Organization of Behavior*, New York: John Wiley & Sons, Inc., 1949.
4. Parsons, T.: *The Social System*, New York: The Free Press of Glencoe, Inc., 1951.

The reality of these multiple systems (General Systems Theory) provides a significantly improved conceptual base upon which to relate new models. The lack of conceptual models able to bridge these divergent systems and allow for action (or intervention) with at least some degree of predictability is a major deficiency in the development of the young science of psychiatry. Social psychiatry represents a legitimate extension of theory formation into systems heretofore neglected, and it cannot come to the attainment of an adequate understanding of the relationship between man and his "world" unless it first becomes actively involved in that world.

At least three systems are involved in the development of so-called social psychiatry. The cultural, social, and psychological systems seem all somehow related, although the conceptual linkages between them are sorely lacking. Despite a probable desire from the reader to have the words social and cultural more adequately defined, this will be avoided. Their definitions are available in the standard works of sociology and anthropology, and at least a global understanding of their meaning (along conventional lines) is probable. The reason for my reluctance relates to my conviction that, whereas a synthesis of social and cultural concepts should redefine our understanding of the psychological, that very synthesis should redefine our concepts regarding the social and cultural. The process of synthesis has mutual impact on all the concepts within the process, hence more than a global definition of social or cultural may be premature at this point. As Bell and Spiegel point out, social psychiatry, as a descriptive term, has an embarrassingly long history.[5] But such an exposé says little about the validity of searching for adequate conceptual models to bring together these three important systems of behavioral determinants. It seems self-evident that such a goal is a worthwhile ideal.

5. Bell, N. W., and Spiegel, J. P.: Social Psychiatry, *Arch Gen Psychiat* 14:337–345, 1966.

There are several directions open to the would-be constructor of models. He may strive to construct a model that is a "candidate for reality," or he may construct a pure model, that is, a model that has meaning with primarily analogous linkages to reality. The former type would hopefully contain linkages beyond the analogous. For example, the psychoanalytic model of mental apparatus (*i.e.* id, ego and superego) is not a candidate for reality since there is no expectation that these constructs exist as such. The model of submolecular particles, however, has a greater relevancy to reality, since instruments have been developed to enable us to describe these particles beyond the analogical level. Besides this hierarchic continuum between reality and pure model, there is model construction relating to action which is based at some level along that continuum. So then, the surgeon whose model of action (or surgical procedure) is based on a model of understanding close to reality acts with less analogical ambiguity than the psychotherapist who acts on the basis of his understanding of models farther removed from reality. Although it is commonly held by science that action models should follow the development of causal models (*i.e.*, treatment based on an understanding of nature), in practice this is only partially possible and often the reverse is the case. The action is often based on less clearly developed concepts regarding cause (less systematic, more a priori, less experimentally validated). Freud's catharsis method preceded his "explanation" of why it helped. Drugs frequently are used before the why of their action is understood. Scientific inquiry makes common use of deductive and a posteriori methodology.

The difficulties which are emerging as more and more turn their attention or criticism towards the renewal of social psychiatry seem based, in great measure, on the failure to differentiate between conceptual models at the various levels of causality and models on the level of action. Much of this is the fault of those involved in establishing programs of social and community psychiatry. They fail to identify goals or to acknowledge their position in the continuum between conjecture and fact. But the critic is as much at fault if he assumes that all interventions are based on an understanding of true nature.

If we turn to the familiar models within psychoanalytic theory, this may be seen more clearly. Psychoanalysis is divisible into a psychological system which attempts to explain behavior, and in so doing provides conceptual models which are helpful in understanding relationships between various identifiable psychologic constructs. Psychoanalysis also provides another level of conceptualization, primarily related to intervention (*i.e.*, treatment) and concepts such as transference, countertransference, resistance, insight through interpretation, etc. operate on this level (action models). The latter level obviously utilizes the concepts of the former, but this should not lead one to conclude a necessary relation between the two levels. It is quite possible that "therapeutic success" resulting from use of the action models of psychoanalytic theory can be explained using causal models bearing no relation to the constructs of psychoanalytic theory. The "explanation" of psychoanalytic success by the school of behaviorists (the conditioning therapies) is such an example. Likewise, the action models of the behaviorists have been "explained" by psychoanalysis using their models, especially of transference and countertransference.

A rather chronic difficulty has been the failure to realize that various causal theories and practices based on the theories have primarily a contingent reality. They exist only in the thoughts of adherents and are of a different order than the realities which are durable and consensually validated. They are only as "real" as they are operationally reliable and predictive. Actions, although commonly linked to "underlying causal" direction, are often really untethered and bear no real relation to their alleged motivation. The explanations for actions commonly develop ad hoc or a posteriori. The point to be made is, although it is to be hoped that causal and action models become related in a real sense, they often spring up unconnected to one another and their linkages may develop erratically, haphazardly, and often backwardly. This is a reality of discovery, and not to be confused with a Baconian preoccupation with inductive scientific experimentation.

Unfortunately, the current attention being paid social psychiatry reflects not only the long-acknowledged need to bridge the psychologic level with the sociocultural, but also the persistent naivete of the panacea makers, who could be deadly in determining the future course of this movement. If the movement is allowed to develop without adequate reflection and understanding of why, it must suffer initial confusion and disorganization, if it develops without an appreciation for its exploratory nature, if it develops with the illusion of being action based on causal understanding, then it will soon be found lacking and the needed multileveled synthesis will again be deferred.

EARLY MULTISYSTEM MODELS

Before discussing the current status and immediate future of social psychiatry, we will briefly comment on selected attempts to provide systems able to bridge beyond the purely psychological level.

If we begin with psychoanalysis we can probably identify the most elaborated system to deal with the task of bridging multiple levels. Perhaps this has more to do with the central position psychoanalysis has enjoyed in psychiatry and less to do with its inherent ability to approach "the whole system." By that I simply mean that psychoanalysis has had more time and manpower dedicated to theoretical elaborations than other theories. The concepts which provide the multilevel bridge in psychiatry are primarily latter-day developments which can be traced to Freud in his latter positions regarding ego and the consequent development of ego psychology. These latter concepts are so removed from identifiable invariables that the term metapsychology (unquestionably a euphemism for metaphysics) has been used to categorize them. Rapaport[6] has traced this development from the initial id-heavy emphasis of Freud to his latter-day shift of attention to ego, and then to the actual primarily autonomous apparatus of the ego (Hartmann[7]). The subsequent theory of the relative autonomy of the ego (Rapaport) is central to a theoretical psychoanalytic basis for social psychiatry.[8] If all behavior flows ultimately through ego function (regardless of unconscious aspects, conflict, etc), then determinants of ego invariably influence behavior. Since, according to Rapaport's model of relative autonomy, the environment is always active (with id) in influencing ego, it follows that the environment, whether it be conceptualized as social, cultural, or both, must be included in further causal conceptualizations. Unfortunately, the status of these conceptualizations is rather marginal. Erikson is a rather solitary, hopeful exception.[9/10] Cummings and Cummings have also ventured into concepts related to the influences of milieu upon the developing ego.[11] If we then look for models of action based on these models of ego-environment involvement, we can find none. The psychoanalytic models of action are preponderantly for intrapsychic dissection. The degree to which the social psychiatrist can look to psychoanalytic models, then, is restricted to the causal models which are still quite primitive.

6. Rapaport, D.: A Historical Survey of Psychoanalytic Ego Psychology, *Psychol Issues* 1:5–17, 1959.
7. Hartmann, H.: *Ego Psychology and the Problem of Adaptation*, New York: International Universities Press, Inc., 1958.
8. Rapaport, D.: The Theory of Ego Autonomy: A Generalization, *Bull Menninger Clin* 22:13–35, 1958.
9. Erikson, E. H.: *Childhood and Society*, New York: W. W. Norton & Co., Inc., 1950.
10. Erikson, E. H.: Identity and the Life Cycle, *Psychol Issues* 1:18–164, 1959.
11. Cummings, J., and Cummings, E.: *Ego and Milieu; Theory and Practice of Environmental Therapy*, New York: Atherton, 1962.

Having considered our mainstream psychologic system, we now flounder badly in trying to find other systems which deal with psychosociocultural synthesis with causal and action concepts or models. Of course the neofreudians (Sullivan, Adler, Horney, Fromm) all deviated from the psychoanalytic line, precisely because of their realization of the importance of extrapsychic factors. The sullivanian concepts tend to focus on the psycho-psycho relationship, *i.e.*, the mutual impact of a psychologic encounter between two individuals, and so his causal models do not encompass the trilevel expanse which we have noted to be a logical "locale" for social psychiatry.[12] The Horney focus was chiefly psychocultural, and, in fact, moved the theoretical base to a cultural norm which defined individual emotional equilibrium.[13] Causal models from this system are available but essentially ignored, and action models are likewise not in vogue. Similarly, the psychobiologism of Meyer made much of the total impact of environment in the longitudinal development of man's psychologic system, but commands a limited following.[14]

Fromm has dedicated considerable energy to conceptualizing along the psychosociocultural dimension, and his formulations, as psychoanalytic variants, are rich in their explicative or "causal" (in our sense) meaning.[15] Again, the implications for action have not been systematically elaborated and have, with those of the other neofreudians, not made sufficient medical impact. The limited status of these "schools" can be related to American medicine in general, and psychiatry in particular, which are

12. Sullivan, H. S.: "Psychiatry: Introduction To The Study of Interpersonal Relations," in Mullahy, P.: *A Study of Interpersonal Relations*, New York: Grove Press, Inc., 1957.

13. Horney, K.: *Neurosis and Human Growth: The Struggle Toward Self-Realization*, New York: W. W. Norton & Co., Inc. 1950.

14. Meyer, A.: *The Collected Papers of Adolf Meyer*, Baltimore: The Johns Hopkins Press, 1951.

15. Fromm, E.: *Escape From Freedom*, New York: Farrar & Rinehart, 1941.

grounded not only in the scientific ethos but in pragmatic activism as well. They do not readily accommodate non-systematic thought, nor thought which does not lead into systematic intervention or action. As Whitehead has stated, nothing dies quite so readily as an idea (regardless of its clarity) if it is not followed by consequent action.[16] The reaction against "philosophic" theorizing within the medical disciplines is a major force in establishing the essential cleavage between the core position, with their implications for intervention and peripheral "oddities."

Although perhaps not immediately apparent, there can be identified a number of syntonic themes between social psychiatry and existentialism, as the latter is usually considered in its applications to psychiatry.[17] The existentialist makes a great point of separating at least three frames of reference which apply to man. The Umwelt, which is an organic biologic concept, puts man into his passive, reflexive, and adaptive mode, and is at least analogous to more primitive psychoanalytic ideas of the id-pushed organism. The Eigenwelt is a more centrally existential concept which relates to man's subjective awareness of himself and which symbolizes his potential autonomy and his latent capacity for commitment and future directed behavior. There is no clear analogous psychoanalytic concept. The third and most relevant concept, for our purposes at least, is that of the Mitwelt. Here is an appreciation for man's vital relationship with his world. As May warns, this . . . . "is not to be confused with the influence of the group upon the individual, or the 'collective mind,' or the various forms of 'social determinism.' The proper focus of Mitwelt is on relationship. The essence of relationship is that in the encounter both persons are changed."[18]

This rather simple statement is so fundamental to the

16. Whitehead, A. N.: *Science and the Modern World*, New York: The Macmillan Co., 1925.
17. May, R.: *Existence*, New York: Basic Books, Inc., 1958.
18. May, R.: ibid., pp. 62—63.

core of social psychiatry that it cannot be overemphasized. This concept, whether couched in the interpersonal focus of Sullivan, the cultural relativism of Horney, the relative autonomy of Rapaport, or the Mitwelt of existentialism, challenges the static dissection of behavior and introduces a complementarity of forces. Like the inner and outer physiology of Park that nurtured medical ecology,[19] these recurrent concepts break down the omnipotent position of the unitary organism and put the issue of behavioral determinism where it belongs, in the mutuality and interdependence of the organism and his context.

But, as in the other positions, the translations of this kind of causal concept into relevant activism or intervention is obscure and vague. Its philosophic foundation casts it into scientific disrepute, or at best condescending acknowledgement.

We come to a rather predictable conclusion. Although there are several "schools" which have directed some attention to the issue of mutuality of social, cultural, and intrapsychic determinants of behavior, none have progressed substantially into a systematic theory of causal character, and even less has been accomplished in offering concepts regarding intervention.

To return specifically to the fundamental questions which the emergence of social psychiatry and community psychiatry raise: What concepts of cause shall direct action? What current action models are relevant? Should action models proceed despite lack of causal systems?

TOWARDS NEW MODELS

It seems safe to say that at this point adequate conceptualizations of a causal nature are in the distant future. The synthesis of relevant concepts in anthropology, sociology, ecology, and medical psychology awaits the general systems scholar as enormous problems. The blend-

19. Park, R. E.: *Human Communities: The City and Human Ecology*, Glencoe, Ill: The Free Press of Glencoe, Inc., 1952.

ing of worthwhile concepts (once identified as such) from disparate psychological schools, each using idiosyncratic language, further compounds the problem.

On this basis, if action models should follow causal concepts, it would seem that social psychiatry's alter ego, community psychiatry, has come before its proper time. The answer, of course, is, as was noted, that action does not always follow the elaboration of a causal system; it frequently precedes. Emerging systems will be the product of the vicissitudes of therapy and theory, the two frequently operative in isolation of one another.

Granting that intervention need not await development of a broad theory of cause (in the social psychiatric dimension), what rational positions should direct the activities of those intent on intervention, i.e., the social or community psychiatrists? Since the interventionist's realm is in many ways undifferentiated, its gradual development and differentiation should proceed in the direction indicated by ongoing self-scrutiny. Any community psychiatric structure which does not maintain an openness and readiness for change runs the high risk of gradual extinction. The whole movement runs the same risk if it does not maintain the same openness. The risks inherent in static programs and structures which attempt to conform to government guidelines are significant.

Assuming that the social psychiatrist begins with an acknowledgement of general systems relevancy, that he is well grounded in traditional clinical psychiatry, that he can generate a cohort of social scientists, that he can lay claim to significant financial support, and that he can tolerate ambiguity, confusion, and frustration, what should he set about to do? What principles of action are likely to remain to a broad mainstream of developing social psychiatry, yet are unlikely to be self-stultifying? We shall divide the following into three general action categories: the social, the cultural, and the psychologic. Since what we are about is the establishment of open-ended action models, our structures should reflect experimental social actions, cultural actions, and psychologic actions. Besides these three "functional" categories, we shall discuss a "teleological principle" as it relates to ordering our actions.

It must be made explicit at the outset that the field in which our action models must operate must be broader than what has heretofore been the case in the general sense of "mental health" and "mental disease." Since the assumption underlying our search states that social process plays a determining role in individual and mass behavior, it follows that our context or field of action must include the social context, *i.e.*, we must deal with the existent social order, structures, and institutions of the locale involved. Then, although the social psychiatrist may not have a clear theory of why or how he is to function, the social field is a proper area in which to work. The expectation and the justification for this seemingly bewildering mandate are that the particles of data that shall comprise future hypotheses and general theories as they relate to psychosocial equilibria and disequilibria will not be accumulated until the interested observers are in fact working with the proper test tubes. Theories of meaningful causal relationships will not emerge from the cloistered sociologist or the cloistered psychologist or psychiatrist. This carries with it the unavoidable dictum that during the beginning phase of social psychiatry (and that may be a long phase) the context of action will be relatively uncharted, vague, and often seemingly out-of-bounds. These features of obscurity are essential and intrinsic to the problem, and are not arguments against the social psychiatric movement.

To move into culture action models is to move from the "shape of things" to the "style of things."[20] Perhaps even more relevant than in the case of social action models is the issue of locale. By this I mean "the where of things,"— the target community, the "catchment area," etc. The

20. Cox, H.: *The Secular City*, New York: The Macmillan Co., 1965.

social psychiatrist functions within geographic or demographic parameters; hence he works with a culturally definable community. This may be homogeneous or heterogeneous (subcultural), but is nonetheless identifiable in gross parameters. The very act of identifying the culture of the area in more specific terms is a function of the social psychiatrist in concert with the anthropologist. An interesting fact in the development of social psychiatry and of the emerging community mental health centers is their predisposition for lower socio-economic area. If the pure principles underlying a psychosocial synthesis are valid, then the movement and the action should be as relevant to the mental health of the person in Darien, Connecticut as it is to the Harlem dweller. Citing the needs of the latter group, the lack of access to psychiatry and the higher incidence of mental illness, the implications of the Civil Rights Movement, concerns about chronic illness, and renewed urban interest are all valid issues, but relate to a different problem. These are largely issues of manpower and its distribution and should not be confused with a desire to ultimately develop principles of behavioral determinism relevant to all persons. This distinction is not often made, however, and "programs" are developed with an obscure raison d'être. It can be charged that this predisposition may more reflect the degree to which the poor can be manipulated than any inherent scientific or humanitarian motive.

Again, the appreciation of cultural norms of any group will not emerge from armchair assumptions. Open-ended action within the group is required to place the participant observer "where the data are." The utilization of indigenous personnel, as in Reisman's Lincoln Hospital project in New York, provides not only an entrée into relatively closed groups, but also to cultural norms manifested by this personnel.[21] There is considerable study already in

21. Riessman, F.: *New Models for a Treatment Approach to Low Income Clients*, read before the American Orthopsychiatric Association Convention, March, 1963.

process on the culture or life style of the poor. It is probable that behavioral determinants on a "cultural level" are of fundamental significance and often go the core of our causal reductionism. This would be truer when dealing with the more culture-bound groups, such as the Negro-ghetto dweller or the immigrant-ghetto dweller, and perhaps less true with the transculturally mobile, *i.e.*, the urban sophisticate. The use of the term "culture" is very broad, however, so we can also search for the "culture" (perhaps it should be called life style) of the sophisticate as well. So then, what is this "culture" of the assembly-line middle-class worker, and how does it contrast with the "culture" of the white-collar middle-class worker, etc? This identification will be no small task since the life styles or "cultures" of people who live in proximity to one another may be very dissimilar. To expect a homogeneous Negro culture, for example, is obviously naive. Time further complicates the dissection, since people may change from one life style to another over a period of time, hence their behavior moves on various causal planes.

If we can briefly use the unconscious-conscious dichotomy, we may discover that the "social" side of things, *i.e.*, the shape of society, will be closer to the conscious side of determinism, while the "cultural" side of things will move closer to the unconscious. I recognize that the use of the terms "social" and "cultural" are broad and require more adequate definition, but, as stated before, I would defer this task since the ultimate working definitions should go beyond the stereotype concepts which have heretofore been used.

Our action is clearly an exploration and when conceived in those terms, is within the finest tradition of scientific empiricism. It is a search for new units of data, units heretofore only globally acknowledged. If our action is evaluated on the basis of its lack of conceptual clarity, the criticism falls on straw men. It is akin to reprehending the explorer for not knowing what he will find when he moves towards uncharted land. Unless he makes the trip, he will never know; and unless the social psychiatrist becomes enmeshed in the wilderness of social and cultural life, he will never be able to identify it meaningfully and determine its behavioral relevance.

Heretofore the bulk of psychological theory has been reductionistic in approach. Behavior has been related in a retrospective fashion to prior occurrences, and so causal explanations have invariably led to a preoccupation with history. Granting the inestimable value of this scientific mechanism, it has not been as productive for psychology as it has been for the hard sciences, such as physics. This is germane to the new perspective of the social psychiatrist. The reduction of behavior of individuals is monumentally complex, and it follows that the behavior of individuals within the broader set of culture and society will not allow for any simple meaningful reduction.

An analysis of sociocultural phenomena may provide academic understanding, but the goal of the community psychiatrist, intervention (action) in the service of "therapeutic change," will have to deal primarily with current realities and not historical relevancies.

This necessity will provide the core of tension within the movement. Psychiatrists, by virtue of their training bias, are ill equipped to deal teleologically, that is, within the framework of the current and its application to future adaptations. When forced to work within this framework, the psychiatrist is beset with beliefs that what he is doing is second-rate, unscientific, compromised, merely supportive. He yearns for positivism, neat dissections, analyses, and reductions. Furthermore, he is unprepared to deal with action which relates to social or cultural change. Since the latter are fundamentally related to power structures and global issues, they have roots that are susceptible primarily to massive forces, but are not easily susceptible to the discrete actions of a solitary physician. This absorption of the interventionist by large social and cultural forces is frustrating for anyone coming out of the authoritarian background of psychiatric training.

The future of social psychiatry seems to extend in at least two directions. On the one hand, there is a need for the development of causal models with relevance to the influence of sociocultural forces on individual psychology. This is a general systems problem and one which focuses on systems around and beyond the individual, *i.e.*, context, variably defined. The second direction is towards an activism heretofore alien to the psychiatrist. It calls for an immersion in the action of social and cultural life. It defines the laboratory as the real active world around us, and asserts that little will be learned about it until one works within it. Activity in this latter direction will hopefully enable us to develop concepts for the former. And as causal concepts emerge, the action models will change accordingly. Those engaged in action at this point are in the area called community psychiatry. It cannot be overemphasized that community psychiatry must become more than the art of more adequate and equitable distribution of psychiatric services; it must become an instrument of social and cultural dissection which bares new ways of linking these forces with psychologic equilibrium. If social psychiatry becomes identified with community psychiatry, and the latter simply develops a new superstructure for the distribution of "service," then as the service reveals itself as old wine in new bottles, the whole structure will wither.

chapter 9

THE FUTURE:

Be It Ever So Humble

IS THERE ONE?

It is intriguing to think about the future of community mental health as a separate and distinct area of applied behavioral science. That future is currently confused with the tinkerings of the community mental health center movement. If the question were posed—is there a future for the community mental health center?—it might be answered in a very different fashion. There will continue to be professionals who are interested in the influences of society on the individual and they will work and study in a variety of contexts and situations. The community mental health center will equally survive in some form or other, but it runs a high risk of becoming another procrustean service structure which may be as inadequate to its surrounding society as the state mental hospital is to today's society. But despite the uncertainty, one is still left with

the option of plodding ahead and stating his wishes, if not
his predictions for the future. This is a dangerous task for
someone who, in the bulk of this book, has been more
critic than creator. It is no secret that the newly accused
will wring their hands in malevolent anticipation when
they learn that their critic is about to lay his own head on
the block. It is not his duty certainly, but having come this
far, why not? And so it seems reasonable, if not prudent,
to pull together some of the foregoing threads, perhaps
lost in the texture of preceding chapters, and mix them
with new threads to fashion an idealized view of a future
community mental health profession. But let me again try
to be clear. When speaking about a community mental
health profession I have in mind the practice, the art, the
doing and not a separated scientific discipline with idiosyncratic fact, theory and research. As was noted in the preceding chapter, community psychiatry (or more generally,
community mental health) is the applied practice based on
facts, theory and research of any of the behavioral sciences
that help the practitioner understand human behavior.
And it is differentiated from the other practitioners of
behavioral intervention, to the degree that it utilizes information from those behavioral sciences at the social end of
the biologic-social continuum.

Community

We are now having a romance with "community." It
will end when we begin to realize that a romance is not a
substitute for real solutions to societal malaise. The romantic illusion should dissipate by the mid '70's. The
burning questions will remain: how to cope with poverty,
crime, poor education, mal-distribution of goods and services, racism, enforced segregation, and on into the littany
of social ills so dramatically characterized by the chaos of
the '60's. The mental health professions will realize that
their resources, tools, knowledge and energy are inadequate for the major tasks needed to bring some resolution

of those social problems. The plight of the individual and the small group (best exemplified by the family) will be rediscovered. There will be greater unanimity in the goal of bringing service to individuals and families.

The "catchment area" albatross will be around for some time. Territorial acquisitions are not easily removed. But coinciding with this decentralizing trend embodied in the catchment area, is a paradoxial trend towards regionalization, which is only minimally palpable now, but which will probably take on great importance in the next decade. The realization that escape to suburbia must be followed by escape to exurbia will eventually slow down the whole migratory phenomena. As people once learned to congregate in cities for their own sake, they will again learn the need to congregate into regional divisions for their own sake. This trend towards regionalization is centrifugal when viewed from the more provincial perspective of a city or suburb, i.e., it is centralization. If viewed from the broader national perspective, it is decentralization (centripetal) with new unit boundaries.

The catchment area concept then is coming at a time when an opposite centralizing trend is about to have its day on stage. The mix between centralization and decentralization will scramble the catchment area so that the current rigid service package for each catchment area will be replaced by more far flung reciprocal arrangements. This may mean that treatment programs for specific problems will *not* be located in the catchment area of the prospective patient. The treatment programs will exist in the more broadly defined region but will not be reproducible in each catchment area. The wish to have services located near a patient's home will succumb to the practical and economic necessity which rejects duplication and redundancy. This will probably mean that the free market model will continue to be dwarfed by the larger bureaucratic model and the issue of quality service will have lower priority.

Planning

Taking the foregoing into consideration it would seem reasonable for the planner to think in terms of regional projections rather than in terms of catchment area, with its population base of 75,000 to 200,000. This will not be easy since, for the time being at least, he must continue to work within federal and local guidelines that are catchment area oriented. But he can certainly begin to establish long range priorities and he can do this through his approach to the defining of "mental health." As has been the plea in earlier sections of the book he should begin to isolate problems that he wishes to systematically attack. With a categorical approach, he can begin to develop service systems which are specific for that problem and which are organized along the natural history of the problem. This is an approach to provide continuity along the longitudinal markers of specific problems, *e.g.* schizophrenia, alcoholism, mental retardation, affective disorders, etc. The listing of specific problems is made difficult by the fact that our current nomenclatures do not list problems in a way that allows us to conceptualize interventional systems.

That brings us again to an oft-repeated plea. We need a nomenclature that differentiates behavior into discrete units which can serve as guidelines for interventional planning. Although knowledge of etiology is the ultimate resource in planning such a nomenclature and although such knowledge is quite sparse, we nonetheless do act out treatment strategies for certain problems. We need to become more explicit about what treatments are used for what problems. This is, in my estimation, an enormous log jam which can be improved even without all of the etiologic connections for which we so fervently wish.

The planner also needs to be less intrigued with innovation for its own sake. If he can settle on problems that have beginnings and endings he will find that his service approach will make more sense. Despite our grandiose inventiveness it is safe to say that basic high quality medical care with continuity and comprehensiveness has not been delivered except in the most grossly maldistributed way. Equalizing the distribution, as unexciting as that might sound, may be the grandest innovation of all.

Manpower

It is unlikely that in the foreseeable future there will be any appreciable change in manpower resource if by that we mean highly trained professional personnel. The shortage means that we will have to maximize the efficiency of those in the mental health professions and inject new kinds of manpower. The new manpower must be trained in a less expensive and less time consuming way than has been the rule in the mental health fields. This depends on two developments which until now have not been well thought out. Again we go back to the development of a task oriented differentiation of behavioral problems (a new nomenclature). That is the primary task and it will be accomplished through trial and error, and serendipity as well as through more a priori behavioral schema. As a new task oriented differentiation occurs then skills and roles will be clarified and training can proceed. Until then, manpower will be a muddle of confusion and shortage and there will continue to be a corresponding mess in service structures and systems.

The creative potential and research possibilities in this manpower issue are enormous. The practical need plus the focus on behavioral differentiation should excite the mental health professional with research or operational interests.

Comprehensive Service

I do believe that persons will be able to obtain more comprehensive services in the future but not from a single source. The difference will lie in the connectedness between various specialized sources rather than in any fundamental change within a source. The difference will be in the ability to put together various sources in a package designed to fit the idiosyncratic needs of the patient or client. This means greater supervening coordination and means reduction of redundant service and/or inappropriate service. Supervening coordination suggests authoritative coordination and that suggests a governmental role. It is my belief that the greatest crisis of the 70's will occur in the area of public services, including not only the usual such as police, fire control, transportation, communication, sanitation, etc., but also in the more ubiquitous services such as those in education, health and welfare. The autonomy of each service producing agency will be reduced in the interest of coordination and we shall see centralized regulatory and distributive functions which will eventually include medicine as well. I believe this will have an effect on quality of service, improving it in those cases where inefficient planning and management have been high and lowering quality in those cases where mal-distribution has been high (as in medicine).

Patient advocacy will be much more plausible in such an ethos and I believe such a development to be inevitable. The community mental health specialist could anticipate such a development and hence prepare or lead the way. It is more likely that he will be led by the nose, complaining at every opportunity.

Prevention

Our society has developed in its technologic dimension at break-neck speed. The life style we use is greatly determined by the gadgets that surround us. The paradox is that our search for mastery over the physical universe has enabled it, the physical universe, to influence our lives in a much more fundamental way than did the uncontrolled universe with its storms, wild animals, and tribal isolation. The price for technical development is the loss of the simple human transaction. We are now electronically one with our neighbors and the world's peoples, so that we can all see and feel our inequality. We are able to turn our righteous aggression, once directed at the saber-toothed tiger, towards a whole nation of people and hate them well. We can now become so thoroughly confused by the bombardment of data and events, that we cut through the confusing truth, to the reassuring conclusion that something like skin color is at the bottom of our problems. Our human computer brains have been overloaded with input and we cannot sort it, relate it nor act from it. We have sparks and buzzing where there should be information and understanding.

The recoil from this blooming, buzzing confusion is apparent all around us. Every institution is cracking and teetering. Human relations are now experimental and confrontational. The search for sanctuary abounds whether in the hippy commune or in a move to the suburbs. Leaders are inadequate in the face of enormous problems and the result becomes a tug-o'-war between anarchy and oligarchy.

That is the flavor of the community at large. The community psychiatrist, coming of age in an age of turmoil, has a great opportunity to see the dynamic of society and culture determining (to a great extent) the behavior of individuals. The proof of the fundamental premise which identifies his field of interest (that individual behavior is shaped in greater or lesser degree by sociocultural forces) is manifest prima facie everywhere around him. He is also coming of age at a time when his tinkering will have but a small role in shaping society and culture. As in the fundamental frustration of psychotherapy, he will be far more able to understand why, than he is able to do anything about it.

I believe it is futile to select certain behavioral phenomena, generally accepted as being maladaptive or dyssocial, and mount a program designed to prevent those phenomena. It makes much greater sense for us to divert our energies into the development of maximally effective social institutions, *i.e.* effective in accomplishing that which they set out to do. And then let the chips fall where they may . . . . picking up the casualties and trying as best we can to rehabilitate them. The problems of our social institutions today are not that they are the wrong ones but rather that they are no longer doing what they were intended to do. The educational system can't and shouldn't substitute for home and family inadequacies. It should and must primarily educate. It must take into account the environmental reality of the students and design its methodology as best it can to meet the peculiar influences of that environment but that can go only so far. It ultimately reaches a methodologic impasse and should not subsume the role of other critical social institutions.

The job of reordering and strengthening our social institutions belongs to everyone inasmuch as everyone depends on our institutional integrity. But in our professional roles we take on different tasks and it is my belief that the mental health professional must be around to help care for, and rehabilitate if possible, those who have not succeeded in the task of adapting to their personal and/or social reality. They should be preventers only when and if they have knowledge about the cause of that which they hope to prevent.

Clinical Services

I have indicated that priorities should be set so that emergency and out-patient services head the list. But the diversity of these services must be set by their ability to accurately differentiate what they do. Again this is an argument for categorization in developing service structures. Services which are vaguely identified as being for persons with mental disorder are too diffuse in their operation to be seriously considered as part of a comprehensive network of human services. Over and over again . . . . a theme central to this entire book . . . . is the need to begin using new nosologic categories. It can be argued, and it could be the readers complaint, that perhaps the whole flurry of activity in community mental health should slow down or even halt until the nosologic problems are recast. I would not argue against such wisdom.

But given the real world, we know that such backward glances provoke rebuke and it is unlikely we shall slow down or halt. But between retreat and defeat there is still time and I am ultimately optimistic. We can do the nosologic job while still balancing the five service structures.

THE UNIVERSITY AND COMMUNITY MEDICINE

Organized medicine has come under severe scrutiny and criticism in recent years. It is clear that the health needs of society have outstripped medicine's ability to meet those needs. The economics of medical care are so complicated that the ordinary doctor never sees the entire picture very clearly. Solutions are strained through political and economic ideologies and there is much confusion as to the future shape of organized medicine. For some critics and analysts, the problem is simply one of economics and, once that is solved, the problems of health care will be resolved. More careful observers note, however, that there are issues which go beyond the economic and have to do with the complexities of organizing the multiple parts of health services so that they are made efficient and so that they better meet the health needs of society. The reorganization that is implicit in this view will not come suddenly nor will it evolve from a single source. We are just beginning to see the first signs of experimental service structures. The montage that will develop will more clearly fit the medical need, but it will do so in a compromise fashion, pushed, pulled and bent to satisfy the heterogeneous elements involved. Medical need is not simply a function of the poor. It is strung out against economic factors, geographic factors, training and education factors, caste and class factors, scientific factors, competitive factors and the idiosyncratic psychology of everyone involved.

It is inevitable that universities will become very much

involved in this exploration for viable types of medical organization. Some are currently explicitly committed to this search, while still others will be caught up in the inevitable trend. The unfortunate rubric that has been attached to university departments interested in this search is "community medicine." It is unfortunate for many of the same reasons noted in Chapter 1.

That this is occurring in universities is understandable and correct. The developmental stages of structure building are always marked by experimentation and self-scrutiny. It is the role of the university to lead in such work since presumably it possesses a great depth of intellectual resource, and since experimentation is at the core of university identity.

PSYCHOANALYSIS, PHILOSOPHY AND PRAGMATISM

Ever since its beginnings psychiatry has labored under difficult conditions. One of its greatest millstones has been its inability to understand its relationship to philosophy. If we were to survey the leading figures in American psychiatry in the last sixty years, we would probably find that they disavow philosophic interest and would place psychiatry into a "scientific" camp as opposed to "speculative" philosophy. That position is a laudatory one. The problem is that, although we are generally in agreement with the scientific orientation, we have had to *use* a philosophic orientation for the survival of our prestige and we have been unwilling to acknowledge that covert dependence.

Because psychiatry evolved through medicine, it has always had the practical identity of being an art (as well as science). In this sense it has always been expected that psychiatrists would "do something." They are expected to act, to be artists. They are not allowed the luxury of isolated speculation or experimentation except within the academic community. The practitioner must practice. Anyone who sets out to "act" must base his actions on a set of "beliefs," otherwise his actions will be purposeless and random. When those beliefs are supported by the weight of validating research and have proven their durability through time, then the action based upon those beliefs can be termed scientific.

In the area of human behavior, as noted elsewhere, we have a slowly growing body of durable belief, supported by experimental work. That validated belief system, however, is far short of a comprehensive system which could allow for understanding of human behavior in all its variation. But the practitioner is hard put to limit his action to those based on validated principles. The demand for his service reflects demands in multiple areas of human behavior where his validated knowledge is sorely deficient. He is compelled to fill in the gaps. He constructs models of a putative sort, essentially making calculating acts of faith to come up with a usable and practical belief system to order his interventions. That process of calculated construction of assumptions is philosophic. The psychiatrist is partly philosopher despite his bitterest protestations.

The issue is most meaningfully dissected when we consider *how much* of the art is based on philosophy and *how much* on validated experimentation. It is unrealistic to expect that an art as young as psychiatry, which deals with so complicated a phenomenon as human behavior, should be comprehensively ordered by validated experimentation. It is a patchwork at best and primitive in comparison to the "harder" arts within medicine. It also suffers an enormous gap between its scientific sources and its practice. As has been repeatedly stated in this work and in others, psychiatry is largely ignorant of much available scientific information which now rests in the nonpracticing behavioral sciences at the social end.

The philosophy of psychoanalysis, which has gripped American psychiatry for much of this century is being slowly eroded by the incursion of various validated beliefs which in some instances are mutually exclusive to psychoanalytic belief. The demythologizing of the dream, and the influence of extra psychic behavioral determinism are examples of this. But whereas the philosophy of psycho-analysis is being eroded, there can be seen an organic development of a science of behavior which includes certain premises once held by psychoanalysis on more tentative philosophic grounds. That is to say that psychoanalysis has and can provide legitimate hypotheses which will withstand the rigors of validating research. The point is that a broadly applicable *system*, which is what psychoanalysis has been, is still largely philosophic and therefore must always be held quite tentatively.

This whole issue of science and philosophy as considered within the problem of behavioral understanding has significant implications for the future of community mental health. To date, the views of human behavior which have marked the central thrust of the mental health professions have been rather unidimensional. They have generally remained within one level of organization: biologic, psychologic, social, anthropologic, etc. Medicine has traditionally attended to mal-adaptations that have been signaled by the human's internal systems, *i.e.*, fever, leukocytosis, pain, pallor, flushing, and the many other signs and symptoms so familiar to medical clinicians. Psychiatry began in this same fashion but of late, for good or ill, has moved in response to external signals of mal-adaptation and social and community psychiatry can be looked at from this source (although not exclusively).

The hypothetic models for the ordering of community mental health practice are no less necessary than models have been for non-community mental health practice. The interplay between action models and causal models will provide the creative process but not without pain. We are still very much at a philosophic level and still very much cranking out more or less valuable "ways of looking" at behavior. Those who will work at the development of new models must discipline themselves to a brand of mental clarity which is able to cut through the maze of system talk, group talk, community talk, individual talk, dynamic talk, biologic talk and onward into a maze of sophisticated and compartmentalized information—some scientific and some philosophic.

THE KIND OF MAN

During the writing of this manuscript there is occurring what has been described as an excessive cut-back of federal support for the community mental health centers throughout the country. Whether this seriously undermines the centers remains to be seen. If this kind of threat disenchants the would-be community mental health professional to the point where he no longer considers himself "interested" in the field, then he is the wrong kind of man to have been interested in the first place. The degree to which the manpower is drained is certainly related to the availability of funds but if professional identity is also drained by money shortage, then we will have proved our early critics correct in their picture of doctors jumping on a money bandwagon and jumping off as soon as the money evaporates.

There are those who will continue despite the money shortages and there are some who feel that money shortage may be necessary to shake from the field those who do it very little good in the first place. And of course there are those who have been "community psychiatrists" long before any such designation was used. These men worked in multiple contexts and without benefit of a broad identity as is the case when one identifies oneself as "belonging" to this field or that. But now there is an emerging identity, albeit vague and as yet open-ended. It has discernible contours and hopefully some of those contours have been identified in this book.

APPENDIX:

A HISTORICAL SUMMARY OF OUT-PATIENT SERVICES

(PSYCHO-SOCIAL CLINIC) OF THE TEMPLE UNIVERSITY

COMMUNITY MENTAL HEALTH CENTER

The charge to the community mental health centers is to develop the five basic services and to develop them along the lines required for adequate service to the specific populations involved. The degree to which innovations and experimentations with psychiatric service delivery systems is implicit in such a charge challenges program developers and administrators and has resulted in a new wave of experimental programming. The following is an attempt to document with some historical continuity the rapid changes and renovations involved in the development of a psychiatric out-patient service to meet the needs of a lower class population group in a large urban center.

Prior to the actual development of clinical services, we examined the catchment area of North Philadelphia demographically. This dramatized the conceptual problems which many have described as being relevant in the development of an out-patient department designed to serve a low income population group. The 200,000 population which comprises the catchment area of the Temple University Community Mental Health Center is characterized by the highest crime rate in the city, the highest rate of infant mortality, the highest rate of substandard housing, the highest unemployment rate in the community and a continuing list of similar parameters which further document the social chaos. Many have indicated that such chaos is inextricable from the high incidence and prevalence of psychological disorder in such population groups. Actual survey work in the psychiatric hospitals serving the population at large of the city of Philadelphia indicated that the patterns of manpower distribution and the patterns of psychiatric caretaking for this population tended to be limited to in-patient services. Out-patient contact was short range, discontinuous, and apparently unequal to the task of preventing readmission to mental hospitals. The nature of the challenge was further complicated by the continuing lack of satisfactory conceptual criteria which could be used to discriminate the sociocultural determinants of behavior from the more strictly psychologic. It was also clear at this early stage of community appraisal that there was a significant sociocultural gap between the value systems and social norms of the community in general and those of the professional caretakers whose task it was to provide service to that population. The disparity in standards of communication and the action orientation of this population have been commented on frequently with negative implications for the use of the medical, highly verbal, psychiatric model of treatment.

To a very real extent, the degree to which in-patient psychiatric services can be innovative is limited by the confining and structuring influences of the hospital in which the in-patient service is to be provided. The same applies to a lesser extent in the development of models of day-hospital care. The development of emergency psychiatric services, however, and the development of out-patient services can be modified to a significant degree depending upon the manpower resources, the types of manpower talents available, and the idiosyncratic needs of the population to be served. The following historical record of the first three years in a developing out-patient department is in many ways a dramatic example of renovative change. To some, the degree of ongoing modification may seem a sign of lack of adequate goal orientation. To the members of the clinic, however, who were instrumental in fostering the many changes, those changes reflect an ongoing commitment to the development of relevant and successful intervention structures. The hope was that these structures would pay more than lip service to the mandate of providing psychiatric care to an out-patient population very unlike the middle class patient population which has been traditionally focused on and which has so significantly directed the treatment approaches in the past sixty years.

STAGE 1—The Beginning

In the fall of 1966, the Out-patient Clinic began its operations within the general out-patient clinic structure of Temple University Hospital in Philadelphia. The clinic operation was located on the fifth floor of a rather modern building and operated under a rather traditional model, including phone-in appointment, short wait for subsequent intake, and eventual assignment to a psychiatric resident under the supervision of a staff psychiatrist from the personnel of the Mental Health Center. The desire of the psychiatric staff of the Mental Health Center to incorporate and integrate the out-patient services of the Mental Health Center with those of the University was one of the primary motivations in the decision to begin the out-patient operation within the University itself. The desire to expose psychiatric residents to the special problems of this population further supported our wish to make the out-patient operation an integrated one within the usual structures of the clinic.

It took only a short time, however, to realize that this program could not succeed in this setting. It quickly became apparent that the psychiatric residents had been oriented toward the evaluation, diagnosis, and treatment of persons whose primary symptomatology and complaints remained rather discretely within the language of psychological disorder. Patients from our catchment area tended to mix their complaints with the many reality problems which complicated their lives. There was a continuing impression that the treatment of this population was in fact an inferior task and one which was ill-suited for the training of psychiatric residents whose ambition it was to perform more traditional psychotherapy with more traditional patients in more traditional settings. To a great degree, the department's teaching philosophy tended to support this orientation. Residents and staff men alike also felt a significant degree of frustration and they recognized their own inability to respond to the urgency and demands of the patients from this population. It became quickly obvious that, in view of the inadequate preparation of manpower, and because of the obvious manpower short-age—which was becoming more obvious—further changes would be in order. It was also clear, at this early stage of development, that patients themselves were dissatisfied and tended not to return.

STAGE II—Physical Move

Our first attempt to change structures was posited on the assumption that there was a significant restrictive influence associated with the actual performance of clinical duties within the traditional out-patient department. We moved the clinic operation to a series of contiguous row-houses in a nearby neighborhood. Our hopes were that a sufficient change in the physical structure would tend to stimulate patient services both by removing the restrictive influence of the hospital setting and by providing a home-like setting. The other major change in the operation of the clinic was to remove the primary treatment responsibility from the resident level and to fix it at the level of staff professionals including psychiatrists, fellows, psychologists, social workers, and nurses.

For a short while this model of clinical service continued; but certain inevitable issues arose. We had not successfully solved the manpower problem and, although we were not being hampered by a high patient contact rate, it was clear that, if ultimately we were able to increase the amount of patient contact, the number of professionals available to provide treatment would always be a significantly limiting factor. Beyond this manpower distribution problem, it was also clear that, although this group of staff persons was professionally committed to serving this population, they had the same conceptual limitations which had been apparent in the residents of the psychiatric department. Treatment tended to be office bound and a high rate of "no show" continued to plague us. It was shortly after having instituted this second stage of operation that a further alternative arose.

The Consultation and Education Section of the Mental Health Center had been involved for several months in an education program with Mental Health Assistants. This training program and the characteristics of Mental Health Assistants are described elsewhere; but in summary the Mental Health Assistants are indigenous, non-professional persons primarily from the catchment area of North Philadelphia who had been recruited and trained to provide supportive assistance to the emerging psychiatric outpatient services of the Mental Health Center. The original role expectation for this group was similar to that of the Mental Health Assistants used in the Lincoln Hospital Project in New York City, that is, of expeditors. It was at this stage of frustration with the clinic, and with the emergence of a group of Mental Health Assistants who showed certain basic talents which we had been unprepared to expect, that the third stage of clinic innovation was developed.

STAGE III—The Mental Health Assistants

It was decided at this point to utilize the services of Mental Health Assistants in a more ambitious manner than they had been previously. The plan was to use the trained Mental Health Assistants as primary "therapists" under a close system of professional supervision. The responsibilities which were assigned to the Mental Health Assistants under this program included intake, initial evaluation of the patient and/or his family, the institution of supportive and rather directive therapy, a broad emphasis on environmental investigation, including home visiting in most cases, and the general provision of ongoing responsibility for out-patient care throughout the time of contact with the center for any particular patient and/or family.

This bold and ambitious plan met with significant resistance not only from the professional community caretakers (school counselors, social work agencies, etc.) but also from a significant number of professional persons within the Mental Health Center itself. The justification for this use of manpower rested on the realization that exclusive professional service would not be possible in view of distribution patterns of professionals which tended to find them in middle and upper class areas. There was further support in the general realization that the sociocultural value system, which to some degree motivated and controlled the behavior of our population group, was an alien one. Although conceivably understood on an intellectual level, it nonetheless escaped the professional person on that more meaningful level which would be most helpful in the provision of relevant psychological care. Armed with these two rational supports for this radical departure from traditional clinical service, we began in the Spring of 1967 to assign patients directly to Mental Health Assistants with the above expectations. The major concession to professionalism was made with the development of a super-structure of supervision. This allowed for close contact between Mental Health Assistant and a supervising professional, usually either a social worker or psychiatric nurse. Cases, including their evaluation and ongoing support, were carefully reviewed with supervisors who gave general guidelines and direction to the Mental Health Assistants, although at times deferring to the rather intuitive talents of the indigenous person. Psychiatrists and psychiatric fellows were used to provide a further network of supportive psychiatric consultation. This was accomplished through the context of individual case-oriented supervisory sessions with Mental Health Assistants, supervisors, and psychiatrists; and in more traditional case oriented conferences where the teaching implications of various cases were used to generalize for the benefit of the entire Mental Health Assistant group. Emphasis was placed on the development of certain characteristics within the Mental Health Assistants including a growing sensitivity to feelings of others, a development of ability to utilize natural and empathic feelings and support of the natural ability to perceive a problem and develop a means toward its resolution. All of these were reinforced with a more intense education regarding the community, its social agencies, and a general outline of psychopathology in an understandable frame of reference.

This rather drastic innovative restructuring of the clinic persisted from the Spring of 1967 until late Fall of 1967. Throughout those months of experimentation, trial and self-scrutiny, it became apparent that the model held many potential benefits, as well as many difficulties which would have to be corrected. One of the more striking developments was the gradual use by the Mental Health Assistant of a more traditional psychotherapy model of interaction, that is the fifty-minute session spent in the confines of an office with the emphasis somehow resting on the full power of "words." A creeping professionalism seemed to be at work which was on the one hand gratifying, since in fact it was a hope that the Mental Health Assistant role could be formalized and made "semi-professional," but on the other hand disturbing, since some of the basic intuitive talents which we were counting on so heavily at the outset were being subverted.

Beyond this gradual model change we were still faced with the reality of a population group submerged in real and difficult social chaos who came to our clinic with complicated problems and with great feelings of urgency. There was a continuing dissatisfaction on our part since it seemed that our intervention model had really not changed enough to become as relevant to the community as was necessary. And so it was in the setting of continuing frustration, although with the tentative excitement of having developed a manpower arm with great potential, that we turned to the next stage of clinic development.

STAGE IV—Community and Crisis

The development of this stage began in mid October 1967. The decision which guided the organization of Stage IV was based on a belief that two factors would be necessary if the clinic for this population was to be successful. The first factor was that the clinic would have to be truly crisis oriented; and the second was that the clinic would have to operate as much as possible within the actual locus of the community, that is within the context of homes, churches, and within those community institutions that might invite us.

We were convinced that the clinic would have to orient itself to crisis because the community seemed crisis oriented. It was clear that help was sought primarily at the time of imminent disaster and during times of maximum stress and disorganization. To be able to intervene at the time of crisis meant that clinic manpower would have to be organized so as to be maximally responsive in very short order and to possess significant "reaching out potential."

The second factor, that is the functioning of clinical operations in the community proper, followed logically from the focus on crisis intervention but also related to the built-in resistance of the community, developed over many years, against the adequate utilization of health services. Studies of patient contact rates had indicated that the primary areas, from which patients came, tended to correspond to the traditional transportation routes to the hospital. Persons who lived near the Center and yet not within easy walking distance were apparently unwilling to utilize the services of the Center unless at a point of maximum personal or family disorganization.

The specific structures designed to provide crisis intervention and maximum community visiting was a three-level organization as follows: At the "hottest" end of the continuum was a Walk-in Clinic and Emergency Psychiatric Unit. This unit had two aspects, the Walk-in Clinic, as its name implies, was a service designed for those who could not or would not use an appointment system. Patients were seen by a team of professionals: a full-time psychiatrist; a senior nurse; two junior social workers and two Mental Health Assistants. All "walk-in" patients or "emergency patients" were seen by one or more of these team members and an initial evaluation was performed on the spot. If it was felt that the case was one which required maintenance of the patient, for from three to five days in a controlled setting, the patient was referred to the emergency section of the "walk-in emergency" unit. Here there were a total of six holding beds with two seclusion rooms for very disturbed cases, and staffed twenty-four hours per day by rotating staff psychiatrists, and a supporting group of psychiatric technicians. If during the initial evaluation it was felt that the patient did not need to be kept in one of the holding beds, the walk-in team could assume responsibility for that patient for up to twenty-one days. During that period of time the team would do whatever they felt was necessary to return the patient and/or his family to a state of equilibrium. The principles which guided this

14 2

intervention were those developed by Caplan and others in the field of crisis therapy. If it was felt, at the time of initial evaluation, that the problem presented by the patient and/or his family was sufficiently complex to require a probable period of intervention to exceed twenty-one days, the patient would become the responsibility of a "Problem Solving Team" which could maintain patient care responsibility for up to ninety days. This team performed the bulk of its services at the Center or during home visits, or at a church "Satellite Clinic," or in borrowed space wherever it was possible to secure space as near to the patient's home as possible. The presumption was that to bring "help" to the natural environment of the patient would enable him to participate more meaningfully with the team and also would prevent members of the team from falling into the more traditional orientation of verbal exchange which in our experience had led very often to minimal results for this population group. This "Problem Solving Team" was composed of one full-time psychiatrist, a senior social worker, a public health nurse, a junior social worker, and four Mental Health Assistants. Besides receiving cases that were first seen within the Walk-in and Emergency teams operations, they would also see many cases where first contact with the clinic was by telephone inquiry. In these latter instances, the point of initial intake might be in the home whenever possible. The community visiting orientation of this group did not preclude its also seeing patients within the center's buildings. It is important to stress that one of the primary criteria of engagement related to a maximum responsibility of ninety days. Again, the implication was that what could be done with a relatively rapid intervention must be done to the exclusion of a long term commitment which reflected primarily the value system of the caretaker rather than of the would-be patient or client.

The third team within the clinic structure was housed within the Mental Health Center buildings and was de-

signed to care for those patients who fit the usual requirements for "psychotherapy." These were patients who were
sufficiently motivated to come for an extended period of
time, to be seen in the setting of an office.

This team also assumed the responsibility for ongoing
care of all patients who had been discharged from our
in-patient psychiatric services. There was no maximum
time commitment involved in this team's operation and it
was, by definition, oriented to more long term and chronic
care. This team also carried out the bulk of family and
group therapy although by no means exclusively. Family
oriented therapy was also part of the operation of the
crisis team and the problem solving team. This "Extended
Treatment Team" provided the active therapy for those
patients at the "coldest" end of the continuum and maintained its connection with the traditional therapies more
so than the aforementioned teams.

STAGE V—Satellite Teams

The three team format (Crisis, Problem Solving and
Extended Treatment) lasted from the Fall of 1967 to the
Fall of 1968. Throughout that period we continued in this
semi-specialized way while gradually becoming aware of
significant handicaps with this type of organization.

The catchment area is sprawling and overly dense. There
is one north-south subway route which can bring patients
to the Center, providing they can easily get to a connecting
station. There is surface transportation along the same
north-south route. Getting to the Center is usually accomplished by taking one of several east-west bus routes
and then transferring to the subway or surface line. Although seemingly a simple procedure, our statistics demonstrated maximum utilization of service by those persons
who lived along the main subway line.

The highest utilization rate of the Center (*i.e.* new admissions to the Center) occurred in the three census tracts
most proximate to the Center. These were rates of 15.2,

12.1 and 11.2 (yearly rate per 1,000 population). Rates varied from 7.6 to 9.8 along the main subway and main surface transportation routes but then fell off in the peripheral census tracts from 6.9 to 3.8 (these statistics derived from figures of May 1, 1967 to April 1968.

This skewing of service use occurred at the expense of high density neighborhoods distant from the subway on the one hand, and the lowest income persons on the other. We attempted to cope with this realization by a total de-centralization of clinic services and the development of six separate satellite clinics located strategically throughout the catchment area. Each satellite had a responsibility for a discrete population (a sub-catchment area) and was to be located in host facilities as these were made available. A host facility was defined as a community-oriented institu-tion which already had stature and relevance in its area and which had invited us to share in its community involvement. ment.

This decentralization was conceptualized as being total so that there would be no centralized out-patient unit with the exception of a small number of clinic administrative personnel who did not provide direct care themselves. Other clinical and non-clinical units were to remain in the centralized series of row homes which had housed the Community Mental Health Center. The Day-Night Hos-pital, the emergency service (Crisis Center), the in-patient beds of Temple Hospital, the consultation and education unit (including community organization), the main record-room of the center, the research group and the overall administration of the Center were all centrally located.

With decentralization there was a corresponding shift towards a generalist approach in each satellite team and we again found ourselves caught by the dilemma of generaliza-tion vs. specialization. The issue of comprehensive care raised other immediate and long-range problems which were made more difficult by our conceptual limitations as well as by the shortage of health care facilities and personnel. The degree to which one either limits or expands the "mental health care" mandate determines the degree to which the Center will be committed to developing its own care resources and to the task of linking with other care-giving institutions. In Philadelphia the shortages of care giving facilities are as profound as anywhere in the country, especially in the areas of mental retardation, alcoholism, geriatrics and addiction. The specialized techniques required for these problems could not be superimposed upon the more basic continuity oriented general service teams which we had developed in our satellite teams.

Although alcoholics represented nearly 10% of new admissions to the Center, they dropped out of treatment generally after their first contact. This well-known phenomenon could only be corrected by a specialized approach to the alcoholic and did not seem vulnerable to correction by a general service team.

Crisis intervention, which heretofore had been provided by a specialized team within our centrally located emergency service (Crisis Center), was to be an integral part of each of the decentralized satellite teams.

We had been impressed by the degree to which our crisis services had been utilized. We were seeing 15 to 20 patients per day (average per twenty-four hours throughout a seven-day week). The commonly held view that low income populations are crisis oriented had been validated in our experience. We were convinced, however, that a centrally located emergency unit tended to attract only the more flagrantly disorganized persons, those whose degree of disability had provoked family, police or community into bringing them to our Crisis Center. We were seeing approximately half of our Crisis Center patients through semi-coercive referral. Of all patients seen in our Center by referral, 54.1% came via police or from the general hospital clinics and only 8.2% were self-referred. We felt that the establishment of a walk-in resource in each satellite would be a significant step towards a comprehensive model of care. We hoped that this development would provide care for a high risk population which was not being served.

STAGE VI—Internal Strife

The reorganization of clinic staff into six satellite teams proceeded despite the lack of host facilities ready to accept the teams. The teams began caring for patients from their sub-catchment areas despite their being housed in the Center. Only one team had succeeded in establishing a true satellite operation and this was in a Church with which we had developed reasonably cordial relations. That satellite had been our pilot operation and its ability to attract patients had been part of the reason for switching the clinic to an all satellite format.

In the midst of developing this decentralized format, which extended from early 1969 through the Summer of 1969, the Community Mental Health Center was experiencing considerable internal upheaval. The Center was beset with disagreement as to its true mandate and split over the clinical services vs social change priorities. Racial charges and counter-charges further polarized staff and there ensued a prolonged period of power struggle and bitter recrimination. The issue of implementation of clinic reorganization was lost in the holocaust and all services tried to hold to the status quo while the broader questions were being debated. Further developments of clinic orientation and organization await the final resolution of a dramatic, and in many ways tragic, identity crisis for the Mental Health Center.

AUTHOR INDEX

SUBJECT INDEX

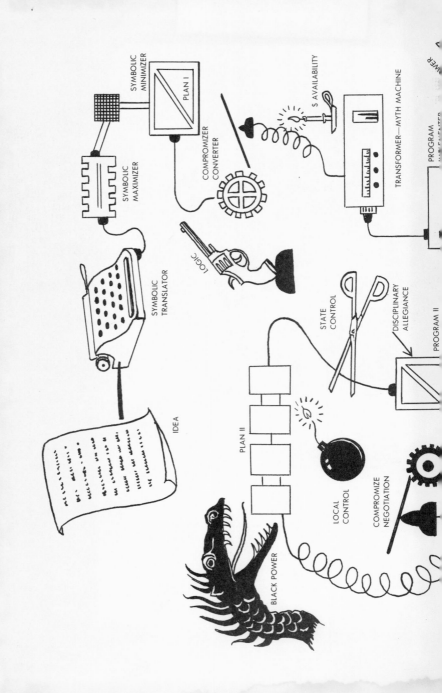